ENCYCLOPAEDIA OF TISSUE CULTURE

Encyclopaedia of
Tissue Culture

Volume 3

M.S. Ahmad

ANMOL PUBLICATIONS PVT. LTD.
NEW DELHI - 110 002 (INDIA)

ANMOL PUBLICATIONS PVT. LTD.
H.O.: 4374/4B, Ansari Road, Darya Ganj,
New Delhi-110 002 (India)
Ph.: 23278000, 23261597

B.O.: No. 1015, Ist Main Road, BSK IIIrd Stage
IIIrd Phase, IIIrd Block
Bangalore - 560 085 (India)
Visit us at: www.anmolpublications.com

Encyclopaedia of Tissue Culture

First Published, 2007

ISBN 81-261-3084-9 (Set)

PRINTED IN INDIA

Printed at Mehra Offset Press, Delhi.

Contents

Preface

A cell is the smallest unit of the body of a living or non-living object. And a combination of cells is called 'tissue'. Tissues are of different kinds and of different shapes and sizes. Some are cylindrical; some are circular; some are long and some others are short in length. Besides, some are soft; some are medium and hard. In common parlance, they form the flesh, blood and bones.

With the advancement in Science and Technology, experiments were also made in this branch of Biology. Replacement of tissues is the major thrust area. Plastic surgery is an example in this connection. With the help of this technology, faces can be changed to any extent. This technology has proved to be a boon for the victims of fire or terrorist attacks.

Like animals, plant tissues also hold a great importance. New to newer experiments are being made at different botanical labs to increase the produce of hybrid plants of varied characteristics. It is a bright career-field and a lot has yet to be done in future.

Encyclopaedia of Tissue Culture attempts at bringing all the relevant and uptodate information on this subject. This multi-volume work includes various aspects of tissue culture at length. Students, scholars, academics, doctors and the general readers would find it equally useful and beneficial.

Comments and suggestions sent by sincere readers would be of great importance to us.

— Editor

1

Gene Conversion

The phenomenon of linkage and crossing over in diploid organisms. It may be recalled that chromosome mapping in diploids is mainly done with the help of three point test-crosses. In haploids, detection of linkage and chromosome mapping is facilitated due to several reasons. *Firstly,* since a single allele per locus is present in a haploid, products of recombination can be studied without any complication due to dominance. *Secondly,* the life cycle of certain fungi *e.g. Neurospora* enables us to analyse the products of a single meiosis. *Thirdly,* in fungi like *Neurospora,* meiotic products are linearly arranged in the form of ordered tetrads, so that a distinction can be made between 'first division segregation' and 'second division segregation' permitting detection of crossing over between centromere and a gene.

Tetrad Division

As mentioned above, in some algae and fungi, the products of a single meiosis can be recovered and examined. The products of a single meiosis may consist of four or eight spores, retained in a sac like structure, and are described as a tetrad. Whenever, the products of meiosis consist of eight spores, they result from four meiotic products undergoing a further mitotic division. These groups of eight may be called octads, but for convenience they are also called tetrads, because they represent paired tetrads (Fig.).

The spores derived from meiotic division, whether four or eight, may be enclosed in two different ways. In some species, like *Neurospora* (also *Ustilago)* the spores are arranged in a linear order and are described as linear or ordered tetrads. In these cases the consequences of first and second meiotic division can be inferred from this linear order. In other cases, however, the spores are mixed and do not retain the order, so that they are unable to suggest the consequences of first and second meiotic divisions. These are described as unordered tetrads. A variety of ordered and unordered tetrads are shown in Figure. That the ordered tetrads can be used to map the centromere on linkage map, a facility not possible with unordered tetrads. The mapping of centromere, facilitated by ordered tetrads, is particularly useful because in algae and fungi, where chromosomes are very small, cytological identification of centromere is difficult.

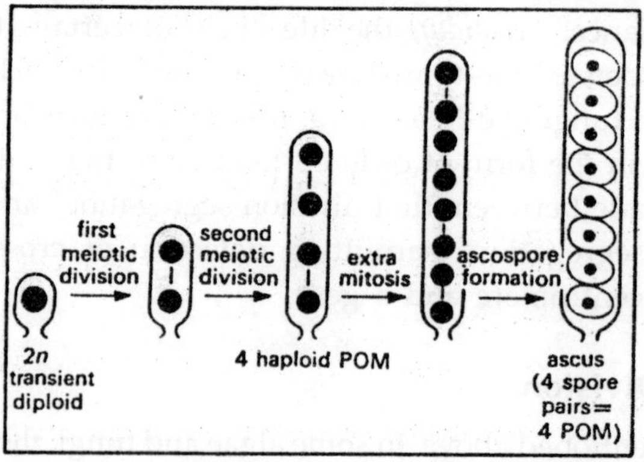

Production of paired tetrad in an ascus, due to linear meiosis and subsequent mitosis (POM = products of meiosis).

The technique of using each of the individual spores of a tetrad for analysis to derive information on linkage and recombination is described as tetrad analysis. Each spore can be separately cultured and its phenotype can be studied to derive information regarding its genotype. For instance, if *A* and *B* are two genes located on different chromosomes, they will undergo independent assortment.

The zygote *AaBb* derived from parents *Ab* and *aB* can give rise to *2Ab* : *2aB* or *2AB* : *2ab* segregation. When the products of meiosis are of only two types, these would be parental ditype (PD) or non-parental ditype (NPD) depending upon whether or not they resemble parents. These parental ditype and the non-parental ditype result due to independent assortment (Figs.). On the other hand, the four products of meiosis from *AaBb* may also be obtained in a ratio *1AB* : *1Ab* : *1aB* : *1ab* thus giving rise to tetratype tetrads, which will result due to crossing over between the centromere and one of the two genes in question (Fig.).

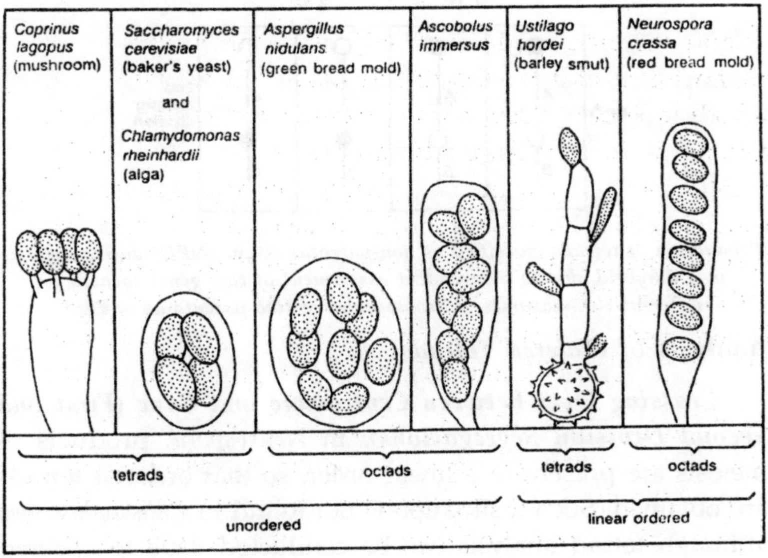

Various forms of tetrads and octads.

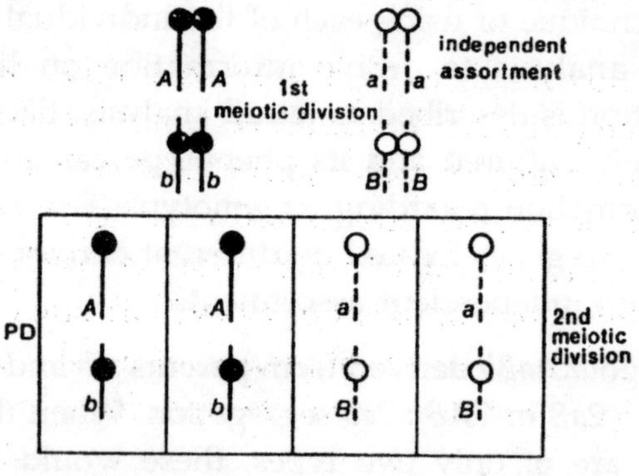

Production of tetrads classified as parental ditype (PD) during meiosis in a dihybrid, due to independent assortment of two genes located on different chromosomes. (Chromosomes of one parent are shown with solid centromeres and continuous lines; those of the other parent shown by empty centromeres and broken lines).

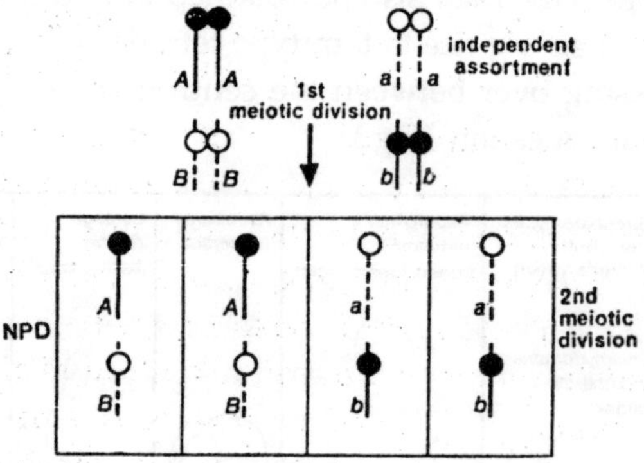

Production of tetrads classified as non-parental ditype (NPD) during meiosis in a dihybrid, due to independent assortment of two genes located on different chromosomes. (Chromosomes of two parents as in Fig.).

Analysis of Ordered Tetrads

Crossing Over between Centromere and Gene (First and Second Division Segregations): In *Neurospora*, products of meiosis are present in a linear order, so that ordered tetrads are obtained. Such a situation is not found in *Chlamydomonas* although tetrad analysis can be conducted. Due to ordered tetrads in *Neurospora*, a cross between normal (a^+) and mutant (a) strain, will give rise to a linear arrangement of four normal spores (a^+) at one end followed by four mutant spores (a) at the other end. Such an arrangement would be disturbed if crossing over occurs between centromere and the gene, because

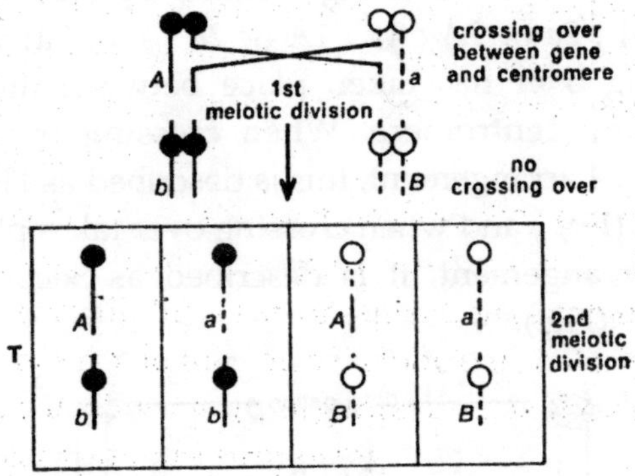

Production of tetrads classified as tetratype (T) during meiosis in a dihybrid, due to independent assortment of two genes located on different chromosomes. (Chromosomes of two parents as in Figure).

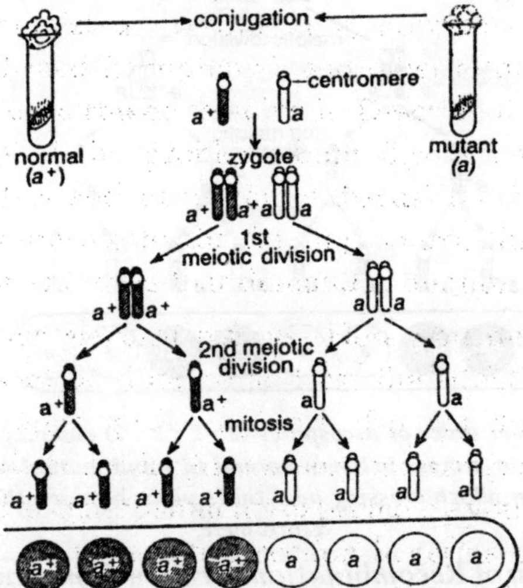

Results showing first division segregation in a cross between normal (a^+) and mutant (a) strains of Neurospora, in which crossing over between the gene and centromere does not take place.

crossing over occurs at four strand and not at two strand stage. If crossing over at two strand stage was possible, it would again lead to four normal spores followed by four mutant spores. Therefore, by analysing linear arrangement, a 4 : 4 arrangement will suggest absence of crossing over and a paired arrangement (*2A* : *2a* : *1A* : *2a* or *2A* : 4a : *1A* or *2a* : 4A : 2a) will suggest that crossing over has taken place between the gene and corresponding centromere. When crossing over is absent leading to 4 : 4 arrangement, this is described as First Division Segregation (Fig.) and when crossing over takes place leading to paired arrangement, it is described as Second Division Segregation. (Fig.).

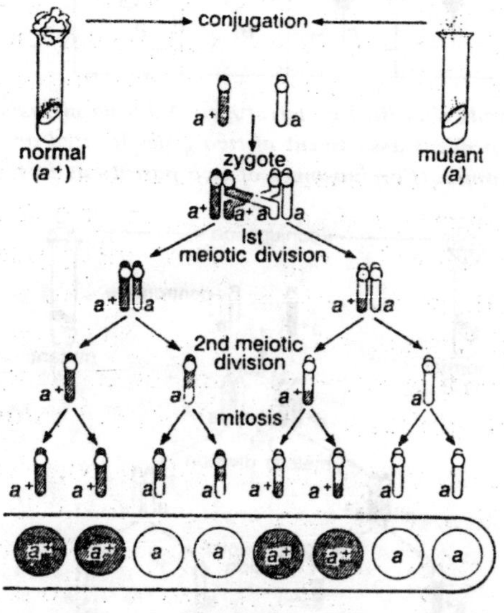

Results of a linear order of ascospores (2 : 2 : 2 : 2) showing second division segregation in a cross between normal (a) and mutant (a) strains of Neurospora, in which crossing over takes place between the gene and the centromere.

Frequency of Recombination between Centromere and Gene: In *Neurospora,* since crossing over between a gene and centromere leads to second division segregation, the relative proportion of asci exhibiting second division segregation will give an estimate of crossing over. This will not be possible in *Chlamydomonas* due to absence of ordered tetrads. As an illustration, in an experiment in *Neurospora,* cross between albino *(al)* and wild type *(al⁺)* gave first division segregation *(al al al⁺ al⁺)* in 129 asci and second division segregation *(al al⁺ al al⁺)* in 141 tetrads. Since only two of the four strands undergo crossing over in second division segregation, recombination between centromere and the gene is,

$$\frac{1}{2}\times\frac{141}{(129+141)} = 0.26 \text{ or } 26 \text{ per cent.}$$

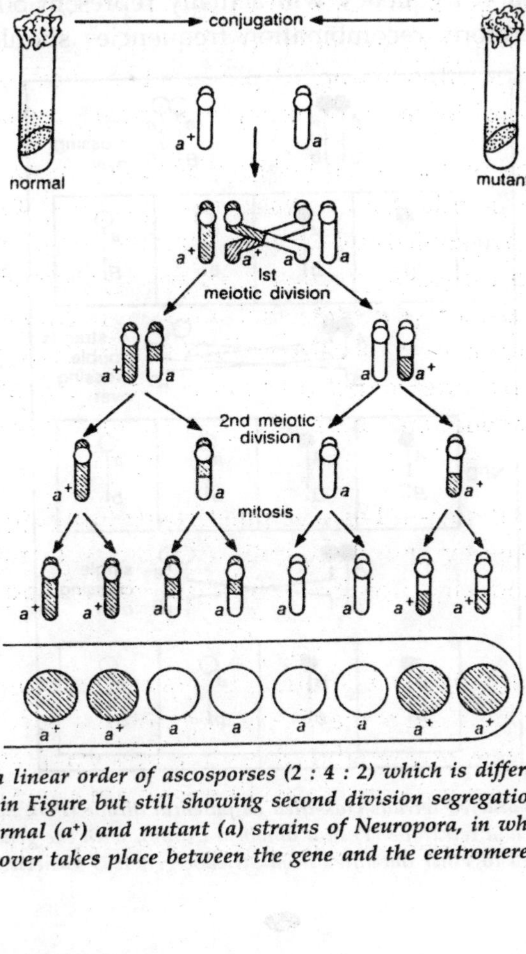

Results of a linear order of ascosporses (2 : 4 : 2) which is different than the one shown in Figure but still showing second division segregation in a cross between normal (a⁺) and mutant (a) strains of Neuropora, in which crossing over takes place between the gene and the centromere.

If a gene is located far away from centromere, crossing over may take place between the gene and centromere in each and every tetrad so that 100% tetrads should exhibit second division segregation. However, since in such cases, double crossovers, and multiple crossovers are also possible, some of the tetrads due to double crossover and other even number of crossover events, will give rise to first division segregation. Thus, second division segregation will never reach 100% level and in practice does not exceed 67% giving rise to only 33% recombination frequency (1/2 x 67, since only two of the four chromatids are involved in crossing over). This 33% recombination frequency will actually represent 50 units or more. Therefore, recombination frequencies should not be

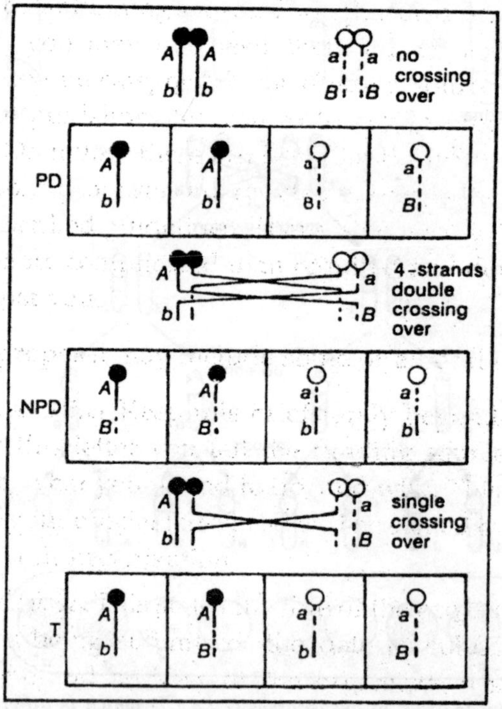

Production of ordered tetrads classified as parental ditype (PD), non-parental ditype (NPD) and tetratype (T) in a dihybrid (AaBb), with the genes A and B linked together (modified from Strickberger, 1977 Genetics).

estimated over long distances, but should be estimated over small distances to avoid underestimation due to double and even multiple crossovers.

Detection of Linkage between Two Genes: We have already discussed that tetrads can be of three types: (i) parental ditype (PD), (ii) non-parental ditype (NPD) and (iii) tetratype (T). The linkage will be detected by comparing your results with the results one would expect on the basis of independent assortment. We have already discussed that if two parents *AB* and *ab* give rise to zygote *AaBb*, it will give PD *(2AB : 1ab)*, NPD *(2Ab : 2aB)* and T *(1AB : 1Ab : 1aB : 1ab)*. If two genes are located on separate chromosomes and independent assortment holds good, PD and NPD tetrads should be equal and T-tetrads should be relatively fewer (since they result due to crossing over in one of the two pairs of chromosomes). On the other hand, if linkage is there, then NPD will result due to four strand double crossovers and tetratype will result due to single crossover, so that the number of NPD tetrads will be much lower, not only in comparison to PD but also in comparison to T (Fig.). This will be illustrated with the help of some data. In *Neurospora*, a cross between an adenine requiring strain *(ad)* of mating type *A* and a wild type strain (+) of mating type *a* gave the results presented in Table.

Results of Tetrad Analysis in a Cross adA × + a in Neurospora (ad = adenine requiring, a = mating type).

Parental ditype (PD)	*Non-parental ditype (NPD)*	*Tetratype (T)*
ad A	*ad a*	*ad a*
ad A	*ad a*	*ad A*
+ *a*	+ *A*	+ *a*
+ *a*	+ *A*	+ *A*
frequency 10	9	1

The data presented in Table can be used for comparing PD and NPD and also for comparing NPD and T. It will be seen that PD and NPD are not significantly different, a result expected only in case of independent assortment. Further, tetratype (T) tetrads are fewer than NPD, a result, which is also expected only from independent assortment, although their frequency relative to the PD or NPD during independent assortrhent will be governed by the distance between the genes and their corresponding centromeres. It can, therefore, be concluded from the data that loci for *ad* and *A* are not linked and are located close to centromere (T tetrads are few). It may be emphasised here that tetrads and not the ascospores or their pairs are considered as units. For instance, if tetrad ratio is 10 PD : 6 NPD, the difference may not be significant, but the ratio of ascospores will be 40 PD : 24 NPD and the ratio of meiotic products will be 80 PD : 48 NPD, the differences in these cases being significant, thus leading us to erroneous conclusion of linkage.

Results of Tetrad Analysis from a cross alA × +a in Neurospora (al = albino; a = mating type).

Parental ditype (PD)	*Non-parental ditype (NPP)*	*Tetratype (T)*		
		1	2	*3*
al A	*al a*	*al a*	*al a*	*al a*
al A	*al a*	*+ a*	*al A*	*+ A*
+ a	*+ A*	*al A*	*+ a*	*al A*
+ a	*+ A*	*+ A*	*+ A*	*+ a*
24	3		27	

In another example of *Neurospora,* an albino strain *(al)* of mating type *A*, and a wild type strain (+) of mating type *a* produced the results shown in Table.

Since in this case, difference between PD (24) and NPD (3) is statistically significant and tetratypes exceed the number of NPD, the data suggest presence of linkage between the two loci.

Preparation of Linkage Map: Data on tetrad analysis can be further utilised for determining linkage distances between genes. Distance between two genes can be sum of the distances of each from the centromere, if they are located on opposite arms or it will be difference of the distances of each gene from centromere if they are on the same arm.

Once linkage is detected, one has to find out whether the two genes are on the same arm or on different arms. The relative frequencies of different orders in tetrads will help in deciding this fact. The different possible ordered tetrads obtained from the cross *AB* × *ab* are given in Table.

In the example used in Table, the two genes are linked *(AB/ab)*. In this case either of the two genes or both the genes may exhibit first division segregation (M_I) or second division segregation (M_{II}).

If the order of loci is centromere-A-B, then the crossing over between A and B will produce M_I segregation for *A* and M_{II} segregation for *B*, as shown in Fig. for tetratype (T) tetrads. On the other hand, crossing over between centromere and *A* will give M_{II} segregation for both and absence Of crossing over in the region 'centromere-A-B' will give M_I segregation for both the genes.

In Table, seven possible classes are given, but the order with in the half ascus was ignored, because it only reflects results of random spindle attachment. For instance PD shown in class 2 in Table, will include all the following four classes, which are equivalent, and can be obtained from each other by inverting top two and/or bottom two genotypes, as expected from random spindle attachment.

AB	*ab*	*AB*	*ab*
ab	*AB*	*ab*	*AB*
AB	*AB*	*ab*	*ab*
ab	*ab*	*AB*	*AB*

The PD, NPD and T types in Table can be obtained by different combinations of M_I and M_{II} segregations *of A* and *B* genes (Fig.). It may be seen that a tetratype can occur only where there is a crossover between atleast one locus and centromere. In other words, for T type tetrads atleast one gene should exhibit M_{II} segregation.

		Bb	
		M_I	M_{II}
Aa	M_I	PD, NPD	Tonly
	M_{II}	T only	T, PD, NPD

The results of first and second division segregations (M_I, M_{II}) for two genes (Aa, Bb), showing that for the production of tetratype (T) tetrads, second division segregation for atleast one of the two genes is necessary.

The distances of two genes from centromeres can be calculated as follows:

$$\text{Centromere-}A = \frac{90+1+5+5}{1000} = \frac{101}{1000} = 10.1\% = 5.05 \text{ m.u.}$$

$$\text{Centromere-}B = \frac{90+1+90+5}{1000} = \frac{186}{1000} = 18.6\% = 9.3 \text{ m.u.}$$

With the above information, following three possibilities exist: (i) *A* and *B* are on two different chromosomes, (ii) *A* and *B* are on two different arms of the same chromosome and (iii) *A* and *B* are on the same arm of a chromosome, *A* lying between the centromere and *B*. The first possibility should lead to independent assortment and can be ruled out, because PD and NPD are not equal and T exceeds NPD. Since M_{II} segregation for both genes exceeds the frequency of a class showing M_{II} segregation for either *A* or *B* alone and since single crossovers will be more frequent than double crossovers, possibility (ii) above is less probable than the possibility (iii), which will give M_{II} segregation for both genes due to single crossover between the centromere and A.

Once it is ascertained that both genes are on the same arm, recombination frequency between *A* and *B* can be calculated. This distance can not be calculated by simple subtraction 9.30 - 5.05, because in calculating 9.30 we ignored double crossovers as in class 6 showing M_I segregation for *B* (Table).

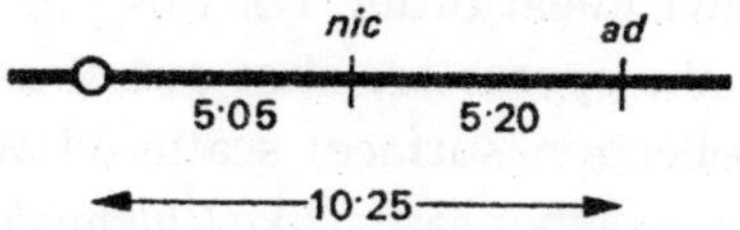

A linkage map of genes A an B based on data presented in Table.

Seven Possible Tetrad Types (with their Frequencies), in a Neurospora Strain Heterozygous at Two Loci (AaBb), Resulting from First and Second Division Segregations (M_I, M_{II}) at either of the two Loci.

Parental ditype (PD)		*Non-parental ditype (NPD)*		*Tetratypc (T)*		
1	*2*	*3*	*4*	*5*	*6*	*7*
AB	AB	Ab	Ab	AB	AB	AB
AB	ab	Ab	a B	Ab	a B	ab
ab	AB	aB	Ab	aB	Ab	Ab
ab	ab	aB	aB	ab	ab	aB
M_IM_I	$M_{II}M_{II}$	M_IM_I	$M_{II}M_{II}$	M_IM_{II}	$M_{II}M_I$	$M_{II}M_{II}$
808	90	1	1	90	5	5

Since all the four products in NPD are recombinants and T has 50% recombinant products, the distance *A-B* can be calculated as follows and a map can be drawn (Fig.).

$$RF = \frac{NPD + \frac{1}{2}T}{\text{total asci}} \times 100$$

$$= \frac{2 + \frac{1}{2}(100)}{1000} \times 100 = 5.2 \text{ m.u.}$$

Analysis of Unordered Tetrads: Isolation of individual spores of a linear tetrad and keeping a record of the linear order of analysed spores is a laborious process. Therefore, sometimes by choice even ordered tetrads are analysed without any record of their linear order. For this purpose, in a fungus like *Neurospora*, the spores are shot out of ascus and may be caught (on a collection surface) scattered without retaining their linear order. In other cases, like *Chlamydomonas, Ascobolus* or yeast, the ordered tetrads are not available and therefore analysis of unordered tetrads is conducted not by choice but by compulsion. In either case, the analysis of unordered tetrads is simpler, though less informative.

The unordered tetrads, like the ordered tetrads discussed earlier, can be classified into PD, NPD and T, although individual tetrads can not be classified as products of first division segregation-and second division segregation. In view of this, although linkage between any two genes can be detected, centromere mapping will not be possible. As discussed earlier for ordered tetrads, the critical test for linkage is the absence of equality between PD and NPD and excess of T relative to NPD. This can be tested by a statistical test (e.g. χ^2 test). This feature is illustrated in Figures, where relationships of the relative frequencies of PD, NPD and T are shown for unlinked and linked loci. It can be shown that the maximum frequency of M_{II} segregation for a gene is 66.7%. When two loci are considered, M_{II} segregation for one locus in combination with M_I segregation for the second locus gives a .maximum frequency of 66.7% for tetratype (T) tetrads. The minimum frequency for either PD or NPD is 16.7. These frequencies hold good for independent assortment. But for linked loci, with increase in the intensity of linkage, frequency of PD increases and the frequencies of NPD and T go down, the frequency of T always remaining higher than NPD. These relationships can be theoretically proved (see Suzuki *et. al.*, 1989 for details).

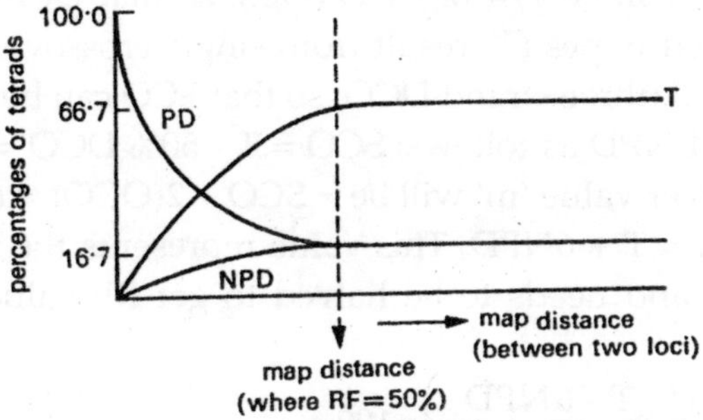

Frequencies of different types of tetrads for linked loci (redrawn from Suzuki et. al., An Introduction to Genetic Analysis 1986).

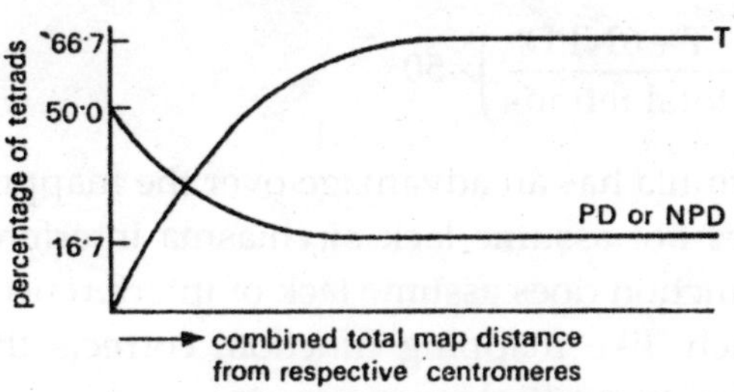

Frequencies of different of tetrads for unliked loci (redrawn frwonm Suzuki et. al., An Introduction to Genetic Analysis, 1986).

As suggested above, if PD = NPD, then RF = 50% indicating independent assortment, but we can not say whether the genes are on different chromosomes or are located distantly apart on same chromosome. In such a situation T type tetrads can be of some use. In an example, where PD = 42, NPD = 48 and T = 10, the tetratype frequency of T = 10 is incompatible with our graph representing linked loci, where T is always more than NPD, and for RF = 50%, T = 66.7%. Therefore, the data suggest that the loci concerned are on separate chromosomes.

It should also be recognised that a maximum frequency of 66.7% for M_{II} gives RF = 33.3% and not the expected 50%. This is due to multiple crossovers. In tetrads, a method is available to correct mapping errors due to double crossovers. If we assume a region having no more than two crossovers or double crossovers (DCO), the NPD resulting from four strand double crossovers, will be 1/4 of DCO (Fig.), so that DCO = 4 NPD. Similarly tetratypes (T) result from single crossovers (SCO) + 50% of DCO (three strand DCO) so that SCO can be calculated from T and NPD as follows: SCO = T - 50% DCO = T -2NPD. The crossover value 'm' will be = SCO + 2(OCO) = (T - 2NPD) + 2(4NPD) = T + 6NPD. This value represents the number of crossovers and needs to be halved to get RF value, so that,

$$RF = \frac{1}{2}\left(\frac{T+6NPD}{\text{total tetrads}}\right)\times 100$$

$$= \left(\frac{T+6NPD}{\text{total tetrads}}\right)\times 50$$

This formula has an advantage over the mapping function since it does not assume lack of chiasma interference, while mapping function does assume lack of interference. However, this approach, like mapping function, corrects the errors in mapping due to multiple crossovers.

Tetrad analysis can also be conducted when three gene differences are involved (for details, consult Strickberger's *Genetics*).

Tetrad Analysis in Higher Plants (A Novel Technology): Since tetrad analysis requires the recovery of all products of a single meiosis, it has not been possible to conduct tetrad analysis in higher eukaryotes. The four products of meiosis in higher eukaryotes either separate from each other, so that products of several meioses are mixed (male meiosis), or they undergo selective death (female meiosis), making it difficult to conduct tetrad analysis. In the year 1998, in *Arabidopsis* (a model higher plant, belonging to the family Crucifereae), quartet *(qrt)* mutation was reported, which causes the four products of meiosis to remain attached. Similar mutants are known in other plants also, although genetic resources like those available in *Arabidopsis* are not available in these other cases thus limiting the utility of tetrad analysis in higher plants to only *Arabidopsis.* These mutants have been utilised for conducting tetrad analysis in *Arabidopsis,* for studies like gamete development, cell division, chromosome dynamics and recombination. In future these mutants will be used for a variety of other studies including gene coversion, not only in *Arabidopsis,* but also in some other plant systems.

Mitotic Recombination and Chromosome Mapping: Mitotic recombination is a phenomenon, which though, first detected in *Drosophila,* has been extensively utilised in *Aspergillus* (a fungus) for detection and measurement of linkage. Therefore, before discussing its nature and utility in *Aspergillus,* the phenomenon of mitotic crossing over, as first discovered in *Drosophila,* will be described in brief.

Somatic Crossing Over in Drosophila: In 1936, Stern studied somatic crossing over between mutants *y* for *yellow body colour* and *sn* for *singed bristles* (bent blunted bristles). Somatic crossing over was inferred from presence of twin spots found in adjacent regions. Crossing over in such somatic tissues has also been found to be enhanced due to presence of genes such as *'minute'*. Let us now consider crossing over in a fly which is heterozygous for both *y* and *sn* genes found in 'trans' configuration or 'repulsion phase' (y +/+ *sn)*. Since it is heterozygous for both the genes which are recessive, only wild phenotype will normally appear (Fig.) except due to somatic crossing over. If the order of genes is *y-sn*-centromere, then following three possibilities of crossing over exist.

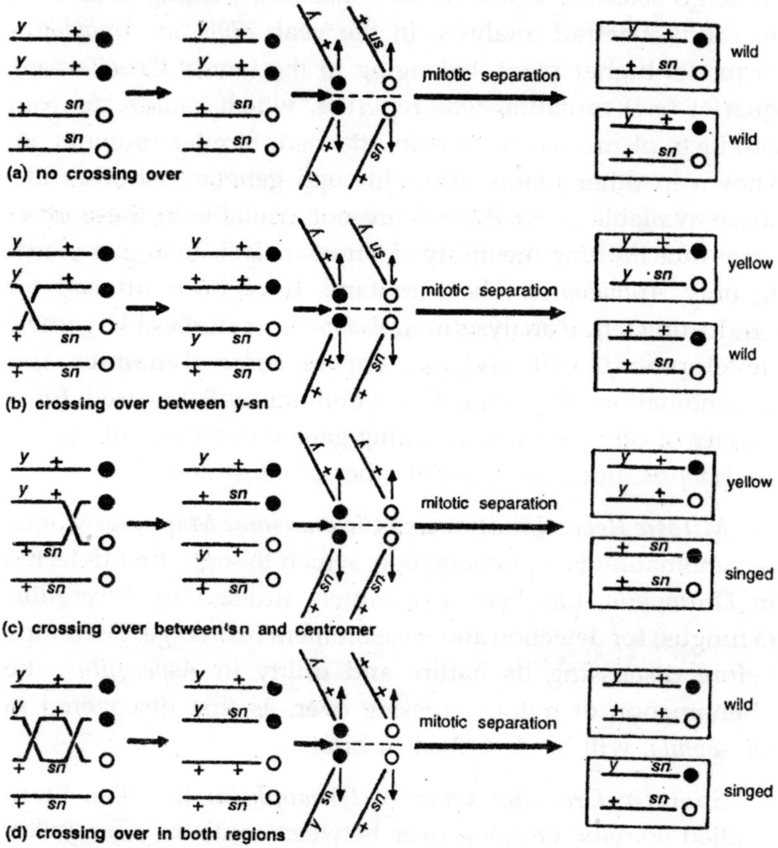

Explanation of results due to normal mitosis and mitotis crossing over in different regions of two X chromosomes of a female Drosophila fly, heterozygous for yellow colour (y) and signed bristles (sn) (modified from strickberger, 1977 Genetics).

Crossing Over between y-sn: As can be seen in Figure B, crossing over between *y-sn* leads to production of two cells with *y+/ysn* (yellow) and + +/+ *sn* (wild) genotypes, so that a single yellow spot will appear wherever crossing over between *y-sn* region occurs.

Crossing over between *sn*-centromere. Crossing over between in-centromere region leads to twin spots, yellow and singed with genotypes *y+/y+* and *+sn/+sn* (Fig.).

Double Crossing Over (y-sn and sn-centromere Regions): Double crossing over results in single spots with singed bristles (y *sn/+sn),* the other product of crossing over giving wild phenotype, i.e. v+/+ + (Fig.).

It was observed by Stern in his study that yellow and singed twin spots were most frequent. This was in agreement with earlier data from meiotic recombination, where it could be shown that the distance between *sn*-centromere is longest and that between *y* and *sn* is relatively very small.

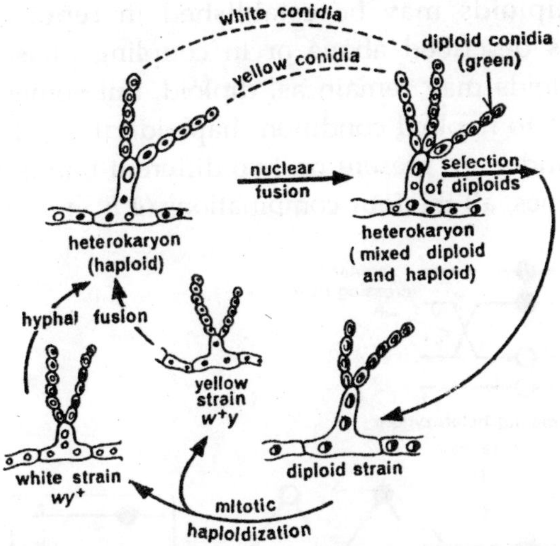

Parasexual cycle in Aspergillus, where diploid formation through heterokaryon and haploid formation without meiotic division are shown. Visible markers in the form of coloured conidia can be used to demonstrate the parasexual cycle.

Mitotic Recombination and Parasexual Cycle in Aspergillus: In *Aspergillus,* like many other fungi, normal vegetative state is haploid. Since mitotic recombination can take place only in presence of homologous chromosomes, a stable diploid condition should first be produced. Diploid strains in *Aspergillus* are often produced due to fusion of nuclei of two strains. In this process, heterokaryons are first produced, where similar haploid nuclei remain separate. These may occasionally fuse to form diploid nuclei, so that both haploid and diploid nuclei will exist and form haploid and diploid conidia, which can sometimes be identified by colour *(white, yellow, green;* Fig.). If two nutritional mutant strains say a (ab^+) and b (a^+b) are used, each will individually need a nutrient for growth and therefore only diploids (ab^+/a^+b) can survive on a minimal medium, not supplemented by any nutrient. Diploid strains can thus be established and characterised by larger conidia and double the DNA content.

The diploids may be established in repulsion phase (ab^+/a^+b) as described above or in coupling phase (ab/a^+b^+). These diploids may remain as, diploid, but sometimes may revert back to haploid condition (haploidisation). In the later case, if a and b are present on two different non-homologous chromosomes, all the four combinations (a^+b^+, a^+b, ab^+, ab) will

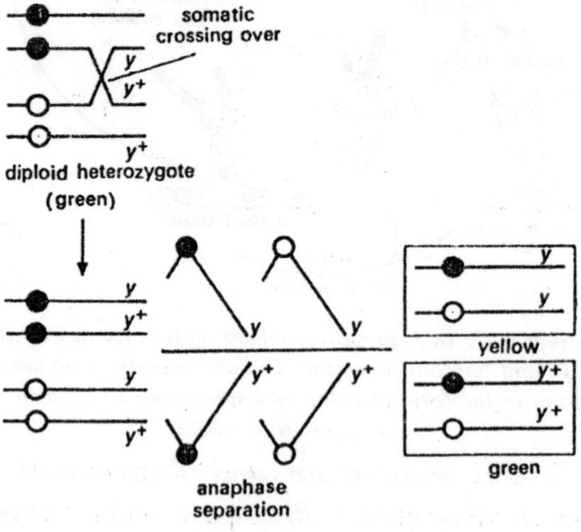

Production of twin spots (yellow and green) due to somatic crossing over in Aspergillus.

be obtained, whether diploid is in coupling phase (a^+b^+/ab) or repulsion phase (a^+b/ab^+). But if '*a*' and '*b*' are located on same chromosome, haploids produced by diploids in coupling phase (a^+b^+/ab) will be mainly a^+b^+ and *ab*, while those produced by diploids in repulsion phase (a^+b/ab^+) will be mainly a^+b and ab^+. By such tests, one can find out whether or not *a* and *b* are linked, because if they are linked, assortment will be non-random (giving two predominant types), otherwise assortment will be random (giving all four types in equal proportions).

The process of haploidisation, may sometimes be accompanied by mitotic crossing over between two linked genes. This may lead to production of recombinant haploids. For instance, if *a* and *b* are linked, diploid (ab^+/a^+b) may also give rise to a^+b^+ and *ab* in addition to ab^+ and a^+b. This process of production of recombinant haploids from diploids has been termed a parasexual cycle, by famous British scientist Pentecorvo. The term *parasexual* has been used since it does not involve sexuality, but produces genetic variability in the same manner as sexual reproduction does.

Since mitotic recombination only rarely occurs during haploidisation, only diploid recombinant products are analysed for chromosome mapping. As earlier discussed, somatic crossing over leads to twin spots. In *Aspergillus* if *y* stands for yellow and is recessive to y^+ (green), then a green diploid (y/y^+) may give twin spots (yellow and green) due to somatic crossing over (Fig.).

Utilizing several markers, diploids heterozygous for different linked markers (e.g. *a, b, c*) may be obtained. A heterozygote $a^+b^+c^+/abc$ may give rise to homozygotes, *aa, bb, cc, aabb, aacc, bbcc* and *aabbcc* in different frequencies. The frequencies will depend on gene order and distances of these markers from centromere. For instance, if the gene order is *centromere-a-b-c*, then *c* -being farthest away will have maximum

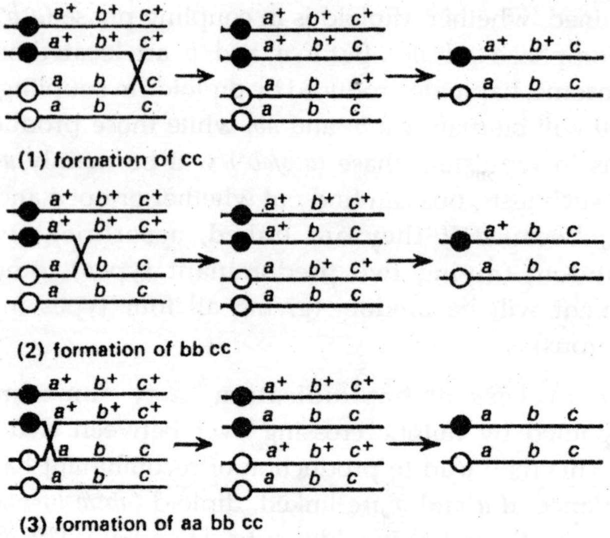

Production of homozygotes cc, bbcc and aabbcc due to somatic crossing over in a heterozygote $a^+ b^+ c^+/abc$, for determining the linear order of genes

likelihood of being obtained in recombinant state ($c/c^+ \rightarrow c/c + c^+/c^+$). If recombinant homozygotes for *c (cc)* are examined for simultaneous homozygosity for *a* and *b* also, three classes can be obtained (Fig.):

(i) *cc* homozygotes which are neither homozygotes for *a*, nor for *b;*

(ii) *cc* homozygotes which are homozygotes for *b* as well, but not for *a, i.e. bbcc* and

(iii) *cc* homozygotes which are homozygotes for *b* and *a* also, *i.e. aabbcc*. This shows that a recombinant for *a* will be homozygote for *b* and c also and similarly a recombinant for *b* will be recombinant for c as well, except in case of rare double crossovers. The reverse is not true, *i.e.* a recombinant for *c (cc)* may not necessarily be a recombinant for *a* or *b*. This kind of relationship among recombinant homozygotes establishes the gene order *a-b-c*.

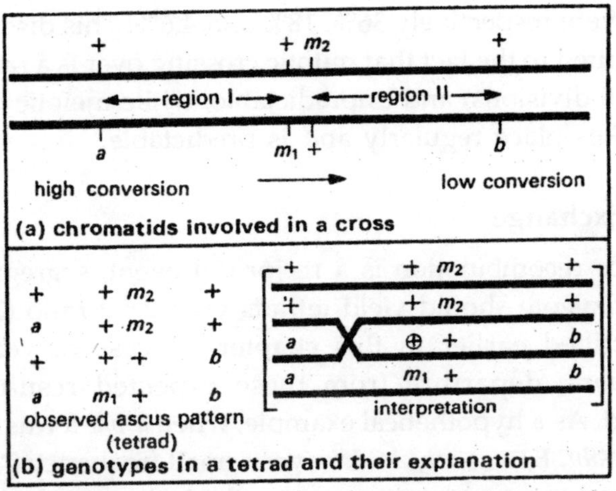

A cross $a^+ m_1 + m_2 b^+ \times a m_1 m_2^+ b$, showing association of gene conversion with crossing over in flanking region; (a) chromatids of a zygote, (b) genetic constitution of a tetrad (conversion $m_1 \rightarrow +$ is accompanied by a crossover between a and m_1, i.e. region I).

Frequencies of the above three classes can be used for estimation of map distances. In *Aspergillus nidulans* three genes, *pro (proline requiring* mutation), *paba (p-aminobenzoate requiring* mutation) and *y (yellow* mutation) were used for preparation of linkage map using mitotic crossing over. Heterozygote $pro^+paba^+y^+/pro\ paba\ y$ gave following results:

(1) *y/y* (crossing over in region *paba-y)*

= 96/371 =26%

(2) *paba-y/paba-y* (crossing over in *pro-paba* region)

= 245/371 = 66%

(3) *pro paba y/pro paba y* (crossing over in *centromere-pro* region)

= 30/371 =8%

It can be seen that recombination frequencies based on mitotic crossing over were 26%, 66% and 8%. These values are different from corresponding meiotic recombination values which were respectively 36%, 18% and 4.6%. This discrepancy is attributed to the fact that mitotic crossing over is a rare event (1 in 100 divisions) and unpredictable, while meiotic crossing over takes place regularly and is predictable.

Gene Exchange

Since recombination is a reciprocal event, segregation in a heterozygote should yield tetrads with 2 : 2 ratio (2A : *2a*) as described earlier in this chapter. In case of yeast and *Neurospora*, departure from these expected results were obtained. As a hypothetical example, when a^+b/a^+b was crossed with ab^+/ab^+, F_1 was a^+b/ab^+. In a very small frequency (4/1000), the recombinant asci, a^+b^+, were available, but their reciprocal recombinant *ab* was not available. Such results could not be explained on the basis of mutations, since the frequency of such events was much higher than expected on the basis of spontaneous mutations, and the event is always directional (in heterozygote $a_1/+$, $a_1 \rightarrow +$, and never $a_1 \rightarrow a_2$). The unusual events were termed gene conversion, a term which was earlier used by Winkler (1930) for an apparent conversion of one gene into another.

During tetrad analysis also, unusual ratios like 6 : 2, 2 : 6, 5 : 3, 3 : 5, etc. were obtained. In these examples, it appears, as if some genes (or alleles) in the cross got converted into the opposite type, without involving any reciprocal exchange event. If gene conversion is a post-meiotic phenomenon, one can assume that 6 : 2 or 2 : 6 ratio will be produced due to conversion of a whole chromatid (both strands of DNA get converted); this phenomena is described as chromatid conversion, as against half chromatid conversion for 5 : 3 or 3 : 5 ratio (only one of the two strands of DNA gets converted).

Some of the properties of gene conversion include the following : (i) There is always a gradient or polarity of conversion frequencies along the gene, if different alleles in a micromap of the gene are considered. In other words, sites closer to one specific end of the micromap show higher frequencies than do those farther away, (ii) Gene conversion of an allele is often (50%) accompanied with crossing over in the flanking regions; this exchange always occurs nearest the allele undergoing gene conversion (Fig.; conversion of m1 involves crossing over in region I and that of m_2 involves crossing over in region II); further the crossing over involves invariably the chromatid involved in gene conversion, (iii) A single conversion event may sometimes involve several alleles of a gene, if the cross is heteroallelic at several sites. This phenomenon is called co-conversion, and its frequency increases with a decrease of distance between alleles undergoing co-conversion.

In view of the above discussion on gene conversion, it is obvious that the phenomenon of recombination includes following two type of events: (i) crossing over, which is a reciprocal exchange of segments and (ii) gene conversion, which is an event involving non-reciprocal transfer of information. Since crossing over and gene conversion differ from each other, we need to find out a possible molecular mechanism of recombination, which should explain both these phenomena. The copy choice theory, earlier described is inadequate for this purpose for reasons described earlier. But several hybrid DNA models have been proposed which explain both crossing over and gene conversion.

2

Genes Synthesised

Molecular manipulation of specific genes is one of the very popular areas of research in biotechnology. These genes, therefore, should be either isolated or artificially synthesised before they are manipulated and used for transformation leading to the production of transgenic plants and animals. Before, we discuss production and uses of these transgenic plants and animals, the gene technology available for isolation, sequencing and synthesis of specific genes should be discussed. This technology will be briefly described in this chapter.

Gene Separation

During 1970's and 1980's, significant progress was made in the techniques for isolation of a variety of genes, including those for:

(i) ribosomal RNA;

(ii) specific protein products;

(iii) phenotypic traits with unknown gene product, and those for;

(iv) regulatory functions *e.g.* promoter genes, etc.

Different techniques have been used for the isolation of these different types of genes and will be briefly described.

Early Attempts for Isolation of Ribosomal RNA Genes in Xenopus

As we know, ribosomes consist of ribosomal RNA (rRNA) and proteins. Ribosomal RNA (rRNA) can be of four sizes namely, 28S, 16S, 5.8S and 5S. This ribosomal RNA makes 80 per cent of cellular RNA and is synthesised on ribosomal genes, which could be isolated. Isolation of ribosomal gene's was considered convenient due to their following three characteristic features:

(i) availability of homogeneous rRNA;

(ii) differences between ribosomal genes and other genes, due to relatively high G+C content in rRNA (rRNA has 45-60% G+C, while the remaining RNA has only 40% G+C);

(iii) ribosomal genes are present in multiple copies, their number within a cell sometimes approaching several thousands.

In view of the above, ribosomal RNA genes were isolated for the first time (as early as 1965, by H. Wallace and M.L. Birnstiel) in an amphibian named *Xenopus*. Following steps were involved in this isolation:

(i) isolate rRNA from ribosomes of *Xenopus* and make it radioactively labelled, due to its replication in a medium containing tritiated uridine;

(ii) isolate ribosomal DNA by density gradient centifugation followed by its denaturation (G+C content of rDNA differs from that of bulk DNA and helps in its separation by centifugation);

(iii) fix single stranded DNA on a filter paper;

(iv) add labelled rRNA on filter paper carrying single stranded DNA;

(v) allow DNA-RNA hybridisation to take place;

(vi) wash excess labelled RNA;

(vii) measure radioactivity and isolate duplex hybrids, which on denaturation, will give single stranded DNA which can then be made double stranded. For a detailed account of isolation of ribosomal genes in *Xenopus* as originally done, readers are referred to an article 'Isolation of Genes' written by Donald D. Brown in Scientific American (August, 1973).

Isolation of Genes coding for known Specific Proteins: Isolation of genes for specific proteins became possible only after the discovery of reverse transcriptase enzyme in 1970. This enzyme can be easily used for the synthesis of copy DNA or complementary DNA (cDNA) from mRNA. This complementary DNA can then be used for the isolation of corresponding gene from genomic DNA. It is therefore obvious that for the isolation of a specific gene, techniques should first be available for the isolation of specific mRNA. For this purpose, antibodies are produced against a specific protein for which the gene is to be isolated. Therefore, isolation of a gene coding for a specific protein involves the following basic steps (Fig.):

(i) purification of the protein product of the gene;

(ii) production of antibodies against this protein product by immunizing animals like rabbit or mouse;

(iii) precipitation of polysomes engaged in synthesizing specific protein with the help of the antibody raised in step (ii);

(iv) isolation and purification of mRNA from the polysome fraction;

(v) using mRNA for synthesizing cDNA with the help of reverse transcriptase;

(vi) cloning of cDNA thus synthesised for preparation of a cDNA library;

(vii) immunological and electrophoretic analysis of the translation products of cDNA clones to identify specific cDNA clone meant for the specific protein in mind;

(viii) use of isolation of gene the specific cDNA probes selected in step (vii) for the identification and isolation of the gene from genomic DNA though screening a complete or partial genomic library for preparation of cDNA and genomic DNA libraries.

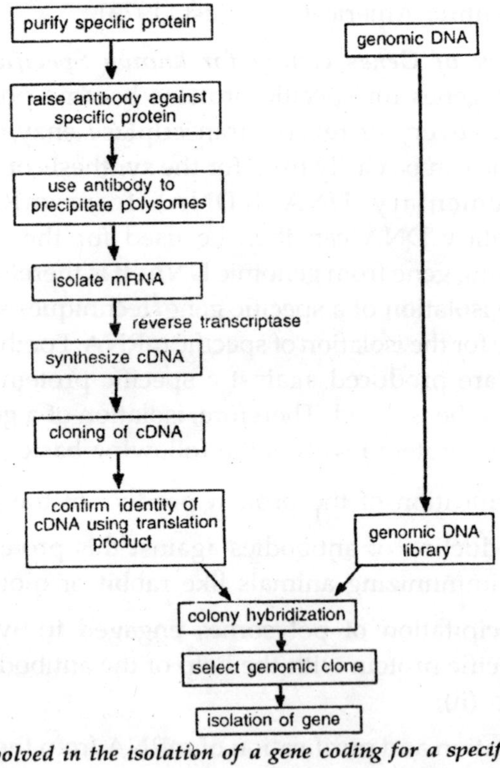

Steps involved in the isolation of a gene coding for a specific protein.

In step (vi) above, for preparation of cDNA library, cDNA may be cloned in expression vectors (vectors in which gene can be expressed due to the presence of promoter sequences for

RNA polymerase enzyme) like λ gt11, which can accept gene inserts into β galactosidase gene. The chimeric vector will then produce hybrid protein if correctly expressed. The hybrid protein can be identified using antibody as above. Plaques belonging to the chimeric vector carrying the desired gene can also be identified by the reaction of the antibody attached to a radioactive protein. The procedure was used to clone a number of genes including a maize gene regulating zein synthesis.

The cDNA clones may also be used directly for gene manipulation and transformation experiments. However, when cDNA clone is used, it should be described as synthesis of gene rather than as isolation of gene, since cDNA has been artificially synthesised, and not isolated from the organism. The above technique for isolation of genes has now been successfully utilised both in plants and animals. However, the first genes isolated were those which existed in multiple copies and were expressed at high level in specific tissues *e.g.* ovalabumin gene in chicks, globin and immunoglobulin genes in mouse, genes for storage proteins in cereals and legumes, amylase genes in barley, actin genes in some legumes, etc.

Isolation of Genes (with known or unknown product), with Tissue Specific Expression

It is much easier to isolate genes which are expressed in specific tissues. For instance, genes for storage proteins are expressed only in developing seeds, ovalbumin gene is expressed in oviduct and globin gene is expressed in erythrocytes. Such genes can be easily isolated because mRNA extracted from these specific tissues will either exclusively belong to the gene of interest or it will be rich in this species of mRNA. Other mRNA molecules in minor quantities can be eliminated, since these can be identified through isolation of mRNA from tissues where this gene is silent. This strategy which is outlined in Figure, was actually followed for isolation and cloning of carrot genes expressed during the development of the somatic embryos, and also in the isolation of several genes for storage proteins in crop plants.

Isolation of Genes (with known or unknown products) using DNA or RNA Probes

Specific molecular probes (whether DNA or RNA probes), if available can be used for isolation of specific genes. These probes may be available either from another plant species or may be artificially synthesised using a part of the amino acid sequence of the protein product of the gene in question.

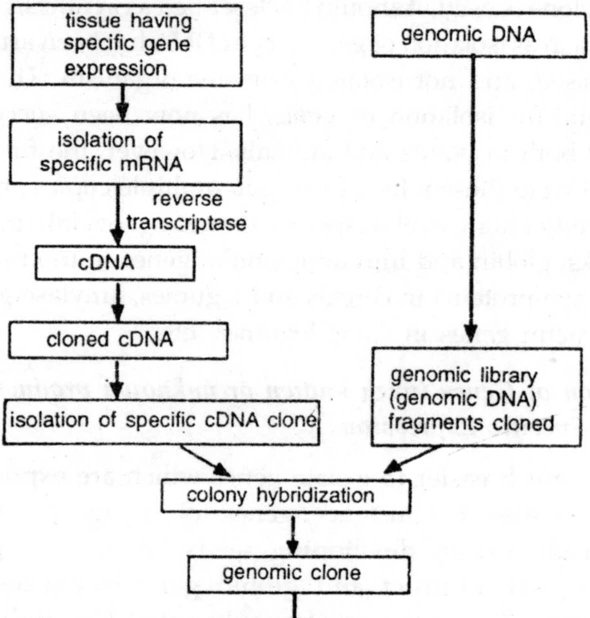

Steps involved in the isolation of a gene with tissue specific expression using its mRNA.

Use of Heterologous Probes: The probes obtained from one plant species and used for another plant species are called heterologous probes. These heterologous probes have been found to be effective in identifying gene clones during colony hybridisation or plaque hybridisation or on Southern blots. For instance, the gene for chalcone synthase (CHS) has been isolated from *Antirrhinum majus* and *Petunia hybrida* using heterologous cDNA probe from parsley. Similarly, heterologous *Antirrhinum* cDNA probe was used for isolation of CHS gene from barley, and heterologous probes from maize were used for isolation of barley genes *Wx* (waxy gene) and *Al* (aleurone gene). Heterologous probes should ordinarily be used with cDNA library and not with the genomic library, since in the latter case, unrelated genes or pseudogenes (which do not express) may be isolated and cloned.

Use of cDNA or Synthetic Probes: We have already discussed the synthesis of cDNA probes above. However, if protein purified using the technique of two dimensional gel electrophoresis, is used for microsequencing of 5-15 consecutive amino acids, this information can be used for the synthesis

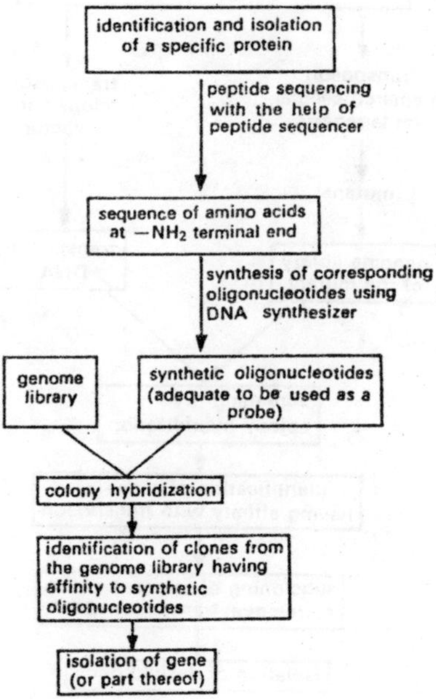

Steps involved in the isolation of a gene using the probe, artificially synthesised on the basis of amino acid sequence of a part of the protein.

of corresponding oligonucleotides (using automated DNA synthesisers). These oligonucleotides may then be directly utilised for screening of cDNA or genomic libraries for isolation of specific genes (Fig.). These can also be used as primers in RT-PCR (reverse transcription-PCR) for the synthesis of cDNA using mRNA isolated from a tissue. A 32 kilodalton (kD) glycoprotein (isolated from style) associated with the S_2 incompatibility allele of *Nicotiana alata,* was used for the synthesis of an oligonucleotide leading to the isolation of a related gene.

Isolation of Genes Coding for an Unknown Product

In some cases, we are interested in isolation of a gene whose phenotypic effect is known, but the gene product has not been identified or can not be isolated. Such genes include

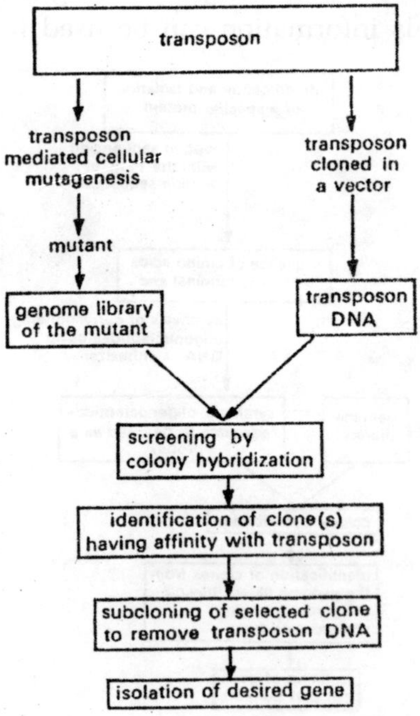

Steps involved in the use of transposon mutagenesis (or tagging) for identification and isolation of a gene.

those for some morphological traits, dormancy, photoperiodicity, disease resistance, etc. This area of research, in which genetics is studied by isolating the gene first without knowing the gene product is often described as reverse genetics. The methods used for the isolation of these genes are different from those used for genes coding for known proteins.

Use of Transposable Elements (Transposon or Gene Tagging): The transposable elements (TEs), in some cases, have been effectively utilised for isolation of genes, when the gene product is unknown. In this case a transposon works as a mutagen and therefore as a gene tag. Following steps which are illustrated in Figure, are involved in this procedure:

(i) A gene with a scorable phenotypic effect is cloned.

(ii) TE is transposed to this gene to get an unstable allele.

(iii) This unstable allele is cloned and TE is isolated from this unstable allele (this is to select a TE which can produce unstable allele).

(iv) This TE is transposed to a gene of interest with known phenotypic effect, to produce unstable allele.

(v) The DNA is extracted from this mutant.

(vi) TE sequence is used as a probe to isolate and clone the mutant gene (carrying inserted TE), so that we can then isolate the gene of interest.

In maize, TE like *Ac/Ds, En/Spm* and *Mul* have been isolated using the genes *Wx, C2* and *Adhl.* These TEs can be used for gene tagging experiments leading to isolation of genes. In maize, several genes like *Bzl, P, Al, Cl* and *C2* have been isolated successfully using gene tagging method.

For gene tagging, often transposable elements endogenous to species like maize and snapdragon have been used. However, rarely transposons available from one plant can be moved into the genome of another plant, whose gene is to be isolated. For instance *Ac* element of maize has been transferred to tobacco, where it can integrate into any locus permitting gene tagging and gene isolation.

Mutant Complementation: In this technique, clones from the wild type strain are selected which should be able to complement the mutants transforming them into wild type. Using these clones, the protoplasts derived from the mutant plant may be transformed and the transgenic plants are produced. Once this is done, the gene of interest can be isolated from DNA extracted from the transformed plants using wild type complementary clone as a probe.

T-DNA Insertion Mutagenesis for Isolation of Plant Genes: A technique similar to transposon tagging is T-DNA insertion for isolation of genes. A limitation of transposon tagging is that it is often confined to either the self fertilized diploid plants such as snapdragon or the cross-fertilized diploid crops like maize, both having well characterised endogenous transposable elements (TE). Although derivatives of maize *Ac* have been successfully used as TE even in crops to which they do not belong, their use is still limited and can not be extended to all plant species. Therefore, T-DNA tagging involving random insertion of T-DNA into the genome, during *Agrobacterium tumefaciens* mediated transformation has been exploited.

The most extensive use of T-DNA insertion mutagenesis has been in *Arabidopsis,* where 35-40% mutations in cultures (used for *Agrobacterium* mediated transformation) were found to be tagged by T-DNA inserts. In 1995, already there were as many as 14,000 transformants, with an average of 1.5 inserts per transformant available at the university of Arizona, Tucson (USA), 40% of them being due to T-DNA insertion. If *Arabidopsis* genome is considered to be 100Mb and T-DNA insertion is random, there is 50% probability for any individual gene to be tagged among the above 14,000 transformants. A number of these genes have been cloned following the steps used for transposon tagging, and are being utilised for improvement of a variety of traits in a number of crop plants.

Since transformants for a large number of traits have already become available, major effort is now needed to isolate any new gene, because a large number of transformed plants will have to be produced and propagated to isolate this new gene. Therefore, if a new gene (for which mutation could not be produced so far through transposon tagging or T-DNA insertion) needs to be isolated, one may like to use a new method to clone the gene of interest.

For instance attachment of a reporter gene to T-DNA will help identification of transformants whenever T-DNA is inserted downstream of a promoter. Similarly attachment of a strong enhancer to T-DNA will allow expression of an otherwise silent gene. This technique permitting identification of transformants may need specific culture conditions and is described as 'enhancer trapping'. In tobacco, this technique has been successfully used for identification of a gene involved in auxin synthesis by growing cultures on a medium not containing auxin.

'Differential Screening'/ 'Differential Display' Technique for Isolation of Genes: A number of genes with unknown gene products are expressed in specialised tissues. Isolation of such genes can be achieved through 'differential screening'. In this technique mRNA is prepared from contrasting tissues of plants such as the following:

(i) tissues/plants exposed to different environmental conditions (*e.g.* drought),

(ii) tissues, which differ in function,

(iii) plants at different developmental stages.

In all these cases, two samples of mRNAs derived from two tissues or two plants should differ and the mRNA species which is not common in both the samples will be identified through differential screening using the following steps:

(i) mRNA is extracted from both tissues/plants separately and used for synthesis of cDNAs using reverse transcriptase;

(ii) cDNAs thus obtained from both samples of mRNA are labelled and used for sequential probing of a genomic DNA library;

(iii) clones that are more strongly hybridised by the cDNA from one mRNA sample than from another contain genes that are differentially expressed in the samples.

One of the limitations of differential screening is that the technique can be used for only those genes that have high expression, and may not prove suitable for those differentially expressed genes that have low expression (low abundance of mRNA). For such genes, another technique called 'differential display' is used. The technique of differential display makes use of polymerase chain reaction (PCR) to amplify rare cDNAs. Following steps are involved (Fig.):

(i) isolate polyA mRNA from two sources as above (call them A and B) and run the following reaction separately with each of the two samples;

(ii) conduct RT-PCR (reverse transcribed-PCR) using as primers 12 possible oligonucleotides of sequence T(11)XY (XY stands for any two of the four bases, thus giving 12 possible dinucleotides); the dinucleotide XY will select the mRNAs, thus providing a means of differential amplification;

(iii) the RT-PCR product is amplified using a pair of primers, one of them being a random 10-mer and the other being the oligonucleotide used earlier in RT-PCR. This will allow amplification of only a fraction of RT-PCR products, including only those to which random 10-mer anneals.

(iv) the PCR products obtained are separated on

polyacrylamide gel electrophoresis (PAGE); it will be noticed that most of the PCR products are present in equal amounts in both samples but some will differ in abundance and still others will be unique in one sample (being absent in the other sample).

(v) the unique bands or the bands showing differential expression are excised and reamplified using the same pair of primers as used in step (iii) above. The reamplified product is cloned and used as a probe for screening cDNA or genomic DNA libraries. Since several genes may have similar patterns of expression in two tissues or two plants sampled, additional criteria will be needed to confirm the identify of isolated gene; this can be achieved by construction of transgenic plants expressing an antisense gene construct.

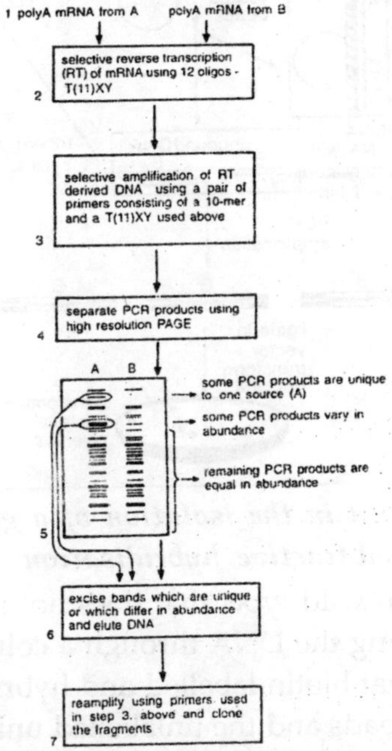

Steps involved in the isolation of a gene using 'differential display technique'.

Subtractive Hybridisation for Gene Isolation: Subtractive hybridisation may help in isolation of a gene for which deletion mutants are available. In this technique, the genomic DNA of wild type may be digested and hybridised by an excess of sheared and biotin labelled DNA from the deletion mutant.

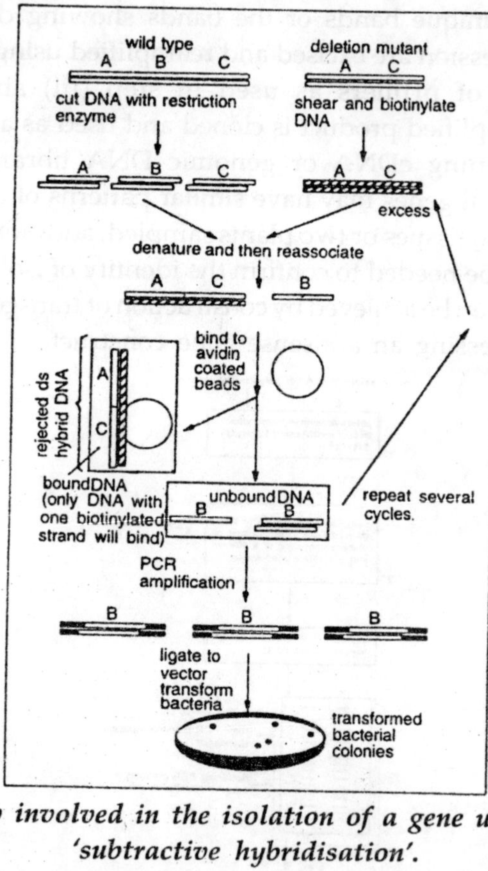

Step involved in the isolation of a gene using 'subtractive hybridisation'.

The DNA from wild type, that does not hybridise, can be separated by passing the DNA through a column with avidin coated beads so that biotin labelled and hybridised DNA will be bound on the beads and the unlabelled unbound DNA will pass out from the column. This process may be repeated through several cycles. The eluted DNA is amplified using

PCR (adapters of known sequences may be labelled and used as primers) and then cloned (Fig.). The clones are then used for hybridisation on the Southern blots of the mutants and wild type to select clones that hybridise only to the wild type and not to mutant type. Further confirmation may be needed to identify the isolated gene.

Map based Cloning of Genes: Map based cloning can be used for isolation of a gene, for which a mutation can be identified, and in a crop for which saturated molecular map is available. Availability of comprehensive genomic library is another requirement. Most of these requirements are now met in all major crop plants. A variety of molecular markers (RFLP, RAPD, SSR or STMS, AFLP, etc.) have been used for the preparation of these maps and can be used for gene isolation. RFLPs will be used here to illustrate the use of molecular markers for map based gene cloning.

(a) *Use of RFLP maps and/or Chromosome Walking for Gene Isolation:* In recent years, RFLP (restriction fragment length polymorphism) maps have been prepared in maize, tomato, rice, etc. Linkage of RFLP loci with genes of interest are also being worked out as an aid to plant breeding. If RFLPs are known which are very close to the target gene (as may be done through RFLP maps and/or chromosome walking), then by locating the RFLPs on either side of the target gene, a long intervening DNA segment or a set of overlapping YAC clones may be isolated. This fragment or the YAC clones (as the case may be) may be used for subcloning, leading to the isolation of the desired gene (Fig.). If RFLPs are examined in two isogenic lines differing for a single specific gene, the difference in RFLP maps of these two lines will help in locating the position of this gene on molecular map which can then be utilised for isolation of the gene. Can also be used for isolation of a gene, if the gene is not far away from the mapped RELP loci.

(b) *Use of Chromosome Jumping for Gene Isolation:* We described the technique of chromosome jumping for walking long chromosome distances, thus bringing the available known sequence (related to the available probe) closer to the gene of interest. Once this has been achieved, the technique may be conveniently used for isolating this gene for further study. The gene for the disease cystic fibrosis in human beings was isolated following this technique.

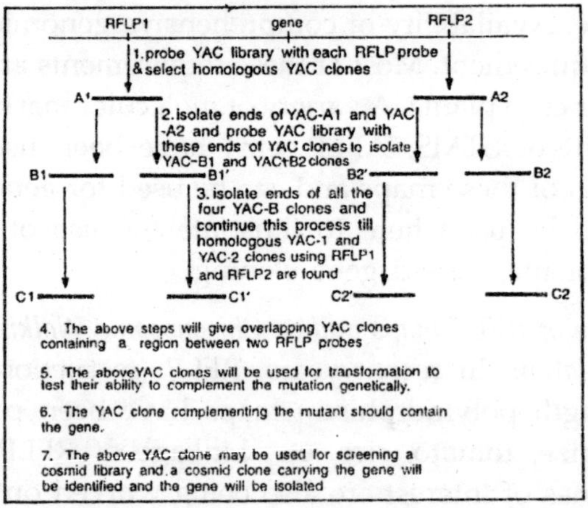

Steps involved in map based cloning, using mapped RFLP loci.

Sequencing of Gene or a DNA Segment: Once a gene or a DNA fragment has been cloned, its further study involves DNA sequencing. The technique of DNA sequencing was very laborious, till 1975, when a breakthrough was made in DNA sequencing methods. Two different methods are now routinely used for determination of DNA sequences.

Maxam and Gilbert's Chemical Degradation Method: In this method, which is illustrated in Figure, following steps are involved:

(i) Lebel the 3' ends of DNA with ^{32}P.

(ii) Separate two strands, both labelled at 3' ends.

(iii) Divide the mixture in four samples, each treated with a different reagent having the property of destroying either only G, or only C, or A and G or T and C. The concentration of reagent is so adjusted that 50% of target base is destroyed, so that fragments of different sizes having ^{32}P are produced.

(iv) Electrophorese each of the four samples in four different lanes of the gel.

(v) Autoradiograph the gel and determine the sequence from positions of bands in four lanes as shown in Figure.

Sanger's Dideoxy Nucleotide Synthetic Method

Frederick Sanger (who won Nobel Prize twice) had initially developed a method for DNA sequencing, which utilised DNA polymerase to extend DNA chain length. This was termed 'plus-minus method'. Subsequently, he developed a more powerful method, utilizing single stranded DNA as template for DNA synthesis, in which 2',3' dideoxy nucleotides (Fig.) were incorporated leading to termination of DNA synthesis. These dideoxy nucleotides are used as triphosphates (ddNTP) and can be incorporated in a growing chain, but they terminate synthesis, since they can not form a phosphodiester bond with next incoming nucleoside triphosphate (dNTP). Following steps are involved in Sanger's dideoxy method for DNA sequencing.

(i) Four reaction tubes are set up, each containing single stranded DNA (cloned in Ml3 phage) or double stranded DNA (cloned in pUC or pBluescript) to be sequenced, all four dNTPs (one of them radioactively labelled) and an enzyme for DNA synthesis (DNA polymerase I; actually a genetically engineered DNA polysase I called 'sequenase' is used due to its high processivity).

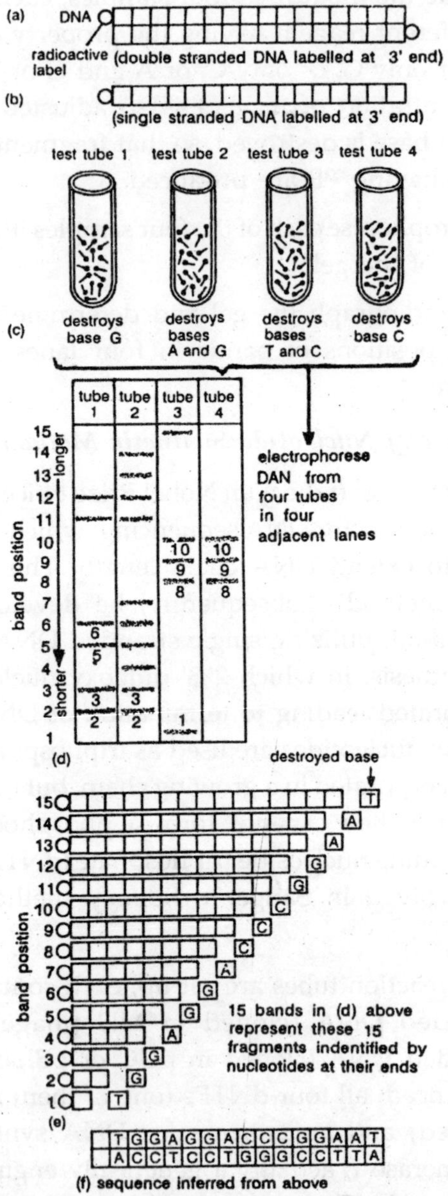

Maxam and Gilbert's chemical degradation method for sequencing of DNA.

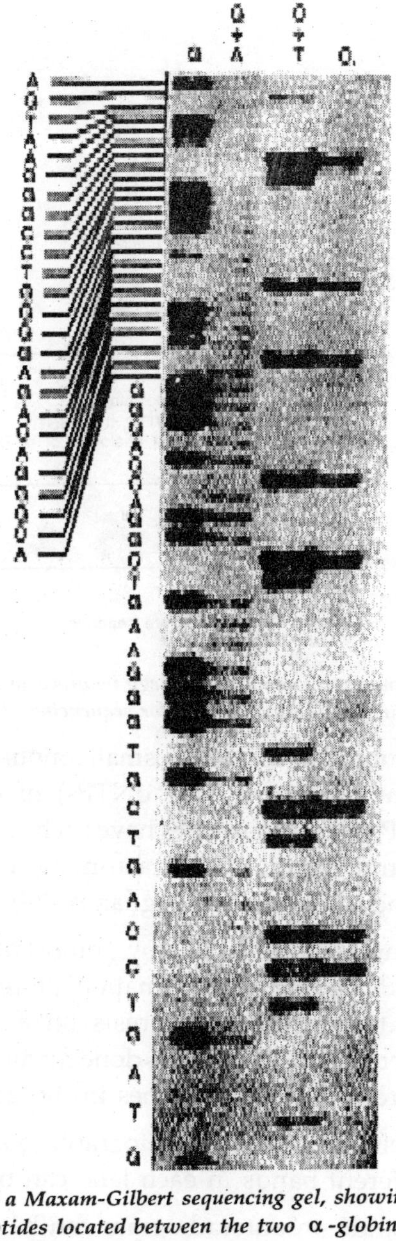

Autoradiograph of a Maxam-Gilbert sequencing gel, showing a portion of a sequence of nucleotides located between the two α-globin genes of human DNA (From, Ayala and Kiger 'Modern genetics 1984)

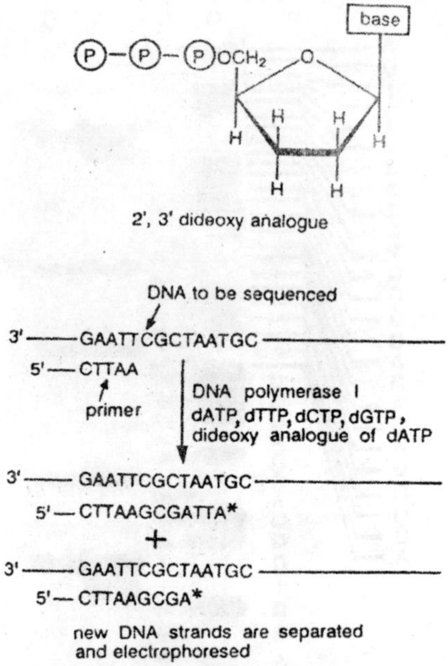

Dideoxynucleotide and the strategy involved in G Sanger's chain termination method for sequencing of DNA.

Each tube also contains a small amount (much smaller amount relative to four dNTPs) of one of the four ddNTP, so that four tubes have each a different ddNTP, bringing about termination at a specific base-adenine (A), cytosine (C), guanine (G) and thymine (T).

(ii) The fragments generated by random incorporation of ddNTP leading to termination of reaction are then separated by electrophoresis on a high resolution polyacrylamide gel. This is done for all the four reaction mixtures on adjoining lanes in the gel.

(iii) The gel is used for autoradiography so that the position of different bands in each lane can be visualised.

(iv) The bands on autoradiogram can be used for getting the DNA sequence as shown in Figure.

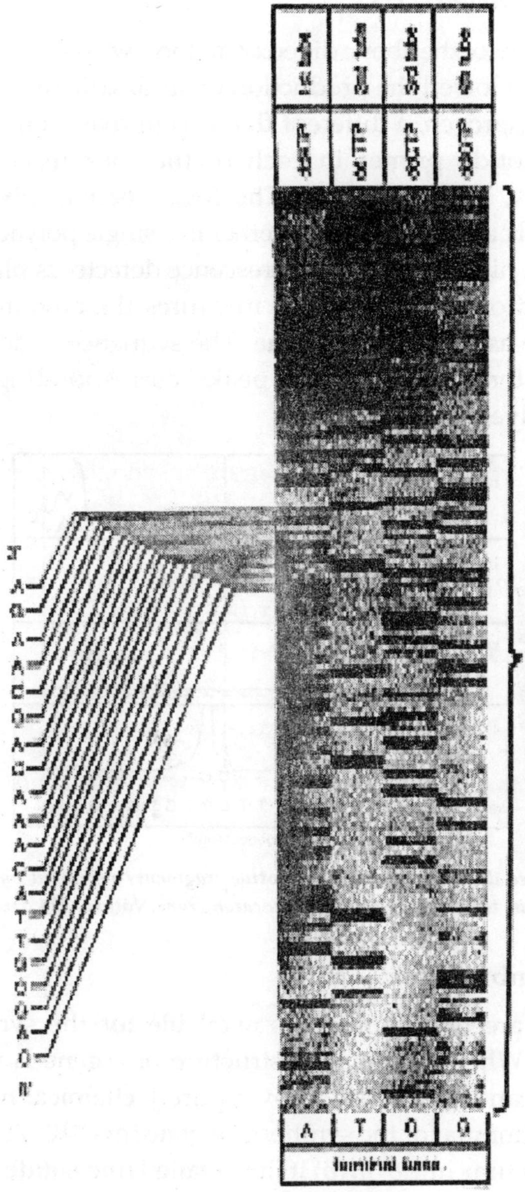

An autoradiograph of Sanger's sequencing gel and the nucleotide sequence read from it.

Automatic Aequencers

A variant of the above dideoxy method was later developed, which has allowed the production of automatic sequencers. In this new approach, a different fluorescent dye is tagged to the oligonucleotide primer in each of the four reaction tubes (blue for A, red for C, etc.). The four reaction mixtures are pooled and electrophoresed together in a single polyacrylamide gel tube. A high sensitivity fluorescence detector is placed near the bottom of the tube, which measures the amount of each fluorphore as a function of time. The sequence is determined from the temporal order of peaks corresponding to four different dyes (Fig.).

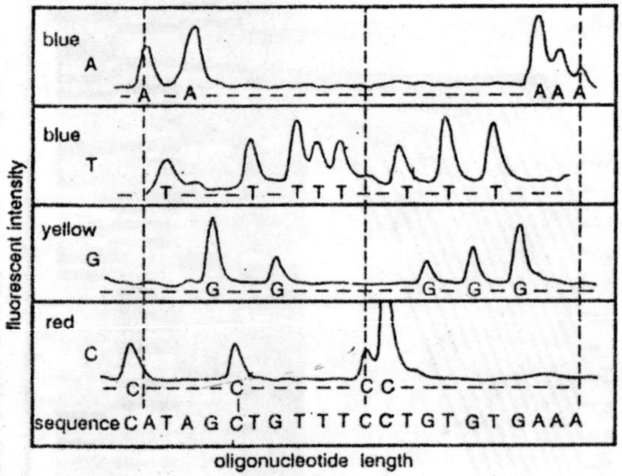

Fluorescence detection of oligonucleotide fragments produced by Sanger's dideoxy chain termination method (redrawn from Nature, 324 : p.674, 1986).

Gene Combination

There are two approaches available for the synthesis of genes: (a) When the detailed structure of a gene is available, this gene can be synthesised by a purely chemical method as done by Khorana for the synthesis of gene for a tRNA (reported for the first time in 1970). (b) If the detailed nucleotide sequence of the gene is not available one may utilise the 'RNA directed DNA polymerase' enzyme for the synthesis of the gene in question in the form of complementary DNA (cDNA) from the mRNA of the gene. As discussed above, cDNA can also be used as a molecular probe for isolation of a gene either: (i) from DNA extracted from living cells utilizing the technique of Southern blot hybridisation, or from (ii) genomic library.

Chemical Synthesis of tRNA Genes

As outlined above, before one can start the chemical synthesis of a gene, the structure of gene should be known. The structure of a gene earlier could not be worked out by direct chemical analysis, since there were no means for isolating a gene. The structure of gene could, therefore, be inferred only from its product. For instance, if a gene is responsible for giving rise to a polypeptide chain and the structure of this chain is known, then from the genetic code dictionary, structure of the gene could be easily inferred (although degeneracy of the genetic code creates problems). Such genes, were initially considered to be too long to be synthesised because an average gene contains about 1,500 base pairs. On the other hand, since tRNA molecules are fairly small in size (about 80 nucleotides), a gene responsible for giving rise to a tRNA molecule was within the reach for artificial synthesis.

Synthesis of Gene for Yeast Alanyl tRNA: The first tRNA whose structure could be known was yeast alanyl tRNA. R.W. Holley (who died in 1993) and his coworkers in 1965 gave a detailed structure of yeast alanyl tRNA (77bp). This information was immediately used by H.G. Khorana and his coworkers to deduce the structure of the gene for yeast alanyl tRNA. The structure of this gene would obviously be such that one of the two strands of DNA (gene) would be complementary to base sequence of yeast alanyl tRNA. The other strand would then automatically have the same sequence as in tRNA except that in place of uracil of tRNA there would be thymine in DNA. Synthesis of such a long chain (77 base pairs) of double stranded DNA was rather difficult in 1965 (not now after more than

30 years) but Khorana and his coworkers had extensive experience of synthesizing DNA of known base sequences. It was decided that such a long chain could not be synthesised by adding a single base each time. Therefore, it was decided that small segments of deoxyribonucleotides ranging in length from 5 to 20 nucleotides should first be synthesised. These segments would be single stranded and would cover the whole length of both the strands of DNA. These would then be joined to form double stranded DNA, 77 nucleotide pairs long. In actual synthesis of yeast alanyl tRNA gene, the following steps were involved.

Synthesis of Oligonucleotides: Fifteen oligonucleotides ranging from pentanucleotide (5 bases) to an icosanucleotide (20 bases) were synthesised. Synthesis was conducted through condensation between hydroxyl group at the 3' position of one nucleotide and phosphate group at 5' position of the second nucleotide. In order to bring about condensation, all other functional groups, not taking part in condensation were protected using specific protective groups. After protecting the groups, reaction between a nucleotide with protected 5' end and another nucleotide with protected 3' end proceed according to Figure. Subsequently codensation was also brought about between groups of two, three or four nucleotides.

Synthesis of Three Duplex Fragments: With the help of 15 oligonucleotides (single stranded), three duplex fragments, each with a single stranded end, were prepared (Fig.). These three fragments consisted of:

(i) the first 20 nucleotides, with the nucleotides 17-20 as single stranded; this fragment was called 'A';

(ii) the nucleotide residues 17-50 with single stranded regions 17-20 and 46-50; this segment was called 'B'; and

(iii) the nucleotides 46-77 with single stranded region 46-50; this segment was called 'C'.

Synthesis of Gene from Three Duplex Fragments: The three fragments 'A', 'B' and 'C were joined to give complete gene in each of the two following ways:

(i) In one scheme, 'A' was joined to 'B' taking advantage of the overlap in residues 17-20; 'C' was then added, with the overlap in the region 46-50 residues. The complete double stranded DNA with 77 base pairs representing the gene was thus ready.

(ii) In the other scheme, 'B' was first added to 'C' and to this 'A' was added in the end to obtain the complete gene. This gene, which was synthesised in 1970, was hopefully used for subsequent work, since this gene could replicate and make its own copies.

Synthesis of Gene for a True Precursor tRNA: Before Khorana could complete the synthesis of gene for yeast alanyl tRNA in 1970, as outlined above, it became obvious that tRNA was not the direct product of transcription. Instead a precursor molecule is first synthesised which subsequently after losing

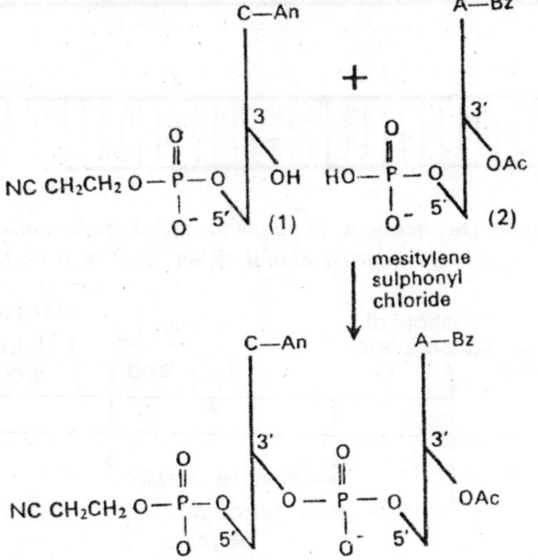

Condensation between two nucleotides with protected 5' PO4 and 3' OH groups in the sugars and protected amino groups in the nitrogenous bases (Ac = acetyl, An = anisoyl and Bz = benzoyl protective groups).

segments of RNA by cleavage, gives rise to tRNA. Obviously, therefore, the actual gene for yeast alanyl tRNA will be longer than the DNA duplex synthesised by Khorana. In view of this, Khorana subsequently initiated synthesis of a gene for *E. coli* tryosine suppressor tRNA precursor.

DNA duplex which will give rise to this tRNA precursor, was synthesised in the form of 26 small oligonucleotide segments. These were then arranged into six DNA duplex fragments having single stranded ends. These six fragments gave rise to presumed gene for *E. coli* tyrosine suppressor tRNA precursor. This gene, however, still lacked promoter region and other sequences essential for processing.

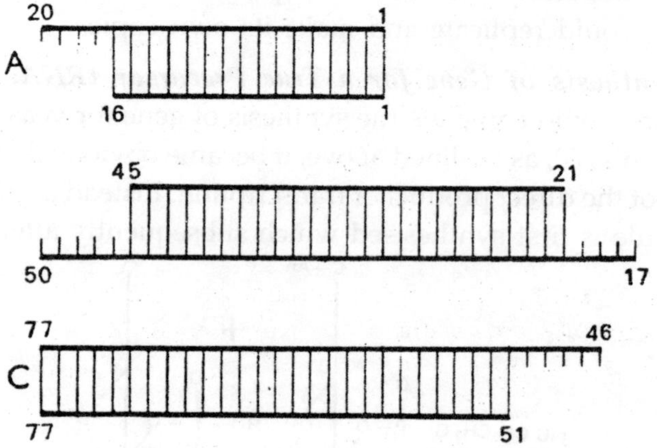

Three duplex fragments, with single stranded sticky ends, produced for the synthesis of yeast alanyl tRNA gene by H.G. Khorana.

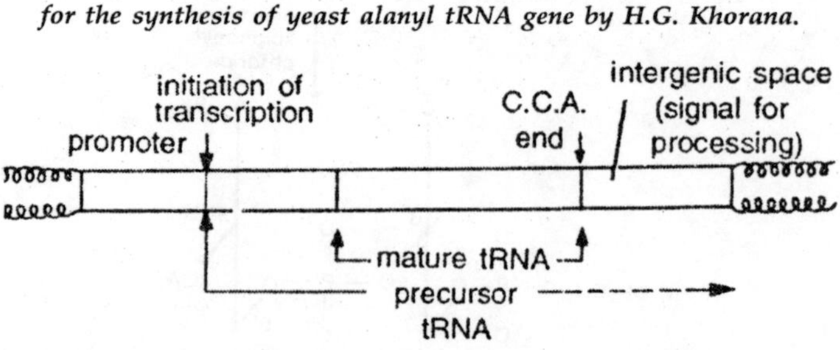

Different parts of the complete E. coli tyrosine suppressor tRNA gene (redrawn from Science, Vol. 203. 1979).

Later, in 1979, Khorana reported completion of the total synthesis of a biologically functional tyrosine suppressor transfer RNA gene carrying all regulatory sequences. This gene was 207 base pairs long and included the following:

(i) a 51 base pairs long DNA promoter region;

(ii) a 126 base pairs long DNA corresponding to the precursor tRNA and

(iii) a 25 base pairs long duplex DNA corresponding to 16 base pairs adjoining CCA end of tRNA and the remainder, a modified sequence including *EcoRl* endonuclease specific sequence.

The details of the complete gene are shown in Figure. The complete synthetic gene was cloned in the vector bacteriophage (lambda virus) by gene cloning method. On transformation of *E. coli,* the phage could multiply with the cloned gene.

Total Synthesis of a Human Leukocyte Interferon Gene

Interferon is a protein, which has a property of inhibiting viral infection and cell proliferation. Therefore, it can be used for treatment of viral infection and malignancies (cancer). These properties have generated great interest in human interferons (IFNs). Atleast three kinds of interferon genes are known in human genome:

(i) leukocyte interferon genes (IFN-α genes),

(ii) fibroblast interferon gene (IFN-β genes) and

(iii) immune interferon gene (IFN-γ genes).

Genes for different kinds of interferons differ and details of base sequences are now known for all of them.

In 1980, Weismann and coworkers published the nucleotide sequence of first IFN-α gene derived from cloned IFN-α cDNA. On the basis of this information, total synthesis of this human leukocyte interferon gene, 514 base pairs long, was achieved and published in 1981 (Edge *et. al.*, 1981). Since there are 514 base pairs in the gene, it involved synthesis of DNA strands with 1028 nucleotides in predetermined way. This was the longest gene synthesised till 1982. The synthesis involved coupling of initial nucleotide on to a polyacrylamide resin to which further nucleotides could be added in pairs. Sixty six (66) oligonucleotide segments varying in size from 14 to 21 were first synthesised, which were then arranged in a predetermined way and joined. This gene has been incorporated into a plasmid and is capable of synthesizing α -interferon. Further details about synthesis of this α -IFN gene are available in the original article published in Nature (Vol. 292, pages 756-761, 1981). The 514 base pairs coded for 166 amino acids = 498 base pairs, and include the initiation and termination signals. There are no intron sequences present in this gene.

The plasmid with this synthesised gene was transferred into bacteria *(E. coli)* which are being utilised now for synthesis of interferon in industry. This has greatly reduced the cost of production of this drug (interferon) which was earlier sold at the rate of Rs. 16 million per 50mg.

Gene Synthesis Machines

Methods for synthesis of DNA molecules of known base sequences have improved dramatically during the last 15 years. Therefore, genes can now be synthesised rapidly and in high yields, sometimes making use of PCR.. For instance, a gene for a tRNA took 20 man years effort during 1965-70, but the same gene can now be synthesised within a matter of few days with the help of a Gene Synthesis Machine. The key innovations which made the availability of gene synthesis machines possible, include the following:

(i) development of silica based supports, which are insoluble and provide support for solid phase synthesis of DNA chains and

(ii) development of stable deoxyribonucleoside phosphoramidites as synthons, which are remarkably stable towards oxidation and hydrolysis and thus are ideal for DNA synthesis.

Several versions of *gene machines* are now available. These machines, under the control of microprocessor, synthesise specific short sequences of single stranded DNA automatically. The desired sequence is entered on a keyboard and the microprocessor automatically opens the valves of the containers of successive nucleotides, reagents and solvents needed at each step, into a synthesiser column, which is packed with tiny silica beads. These beads provide support on which DNA molecules are assembled (Fig.).

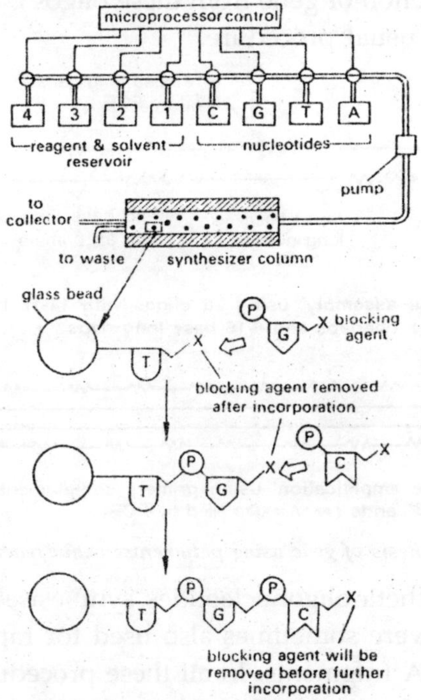

An outline of a gene synthesis machine, which synthesises a gene automatically once the nucleotide sequences are entered in the microprocessor.

Synthesis of Gene Using PCR

The methods of gene synthesis utilised earlier, whether manual or using automatic synthesisers, involved the following steps:

(i) synthesis of oligos,

(ii) annealing of oligos to give duplexes with single stranded cohesive or sticky ends, and

(iii) ligation of duplexes to obtain complete gene.

This strategy was initially used by Khorana and was subsequently followed by many. Even while using automatic synthesisers, only the oligos are synthesised on the synthesiser, but the production of gene from these oligos is achieved later following the usual procedure.

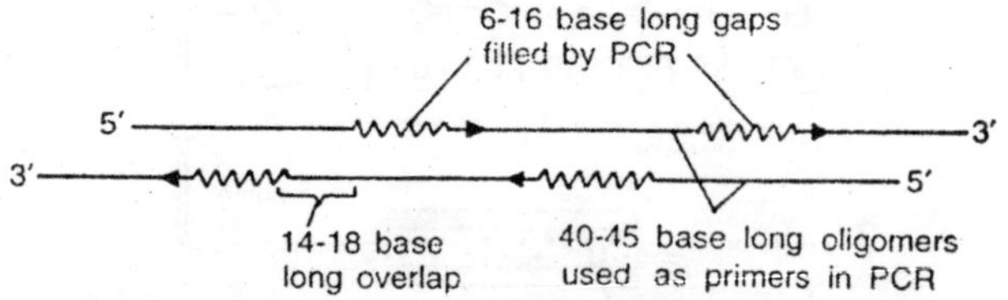

(a) 'gene assembly' using 28 oligos with 14-18 base long overlaps and 6-16 base long gaps

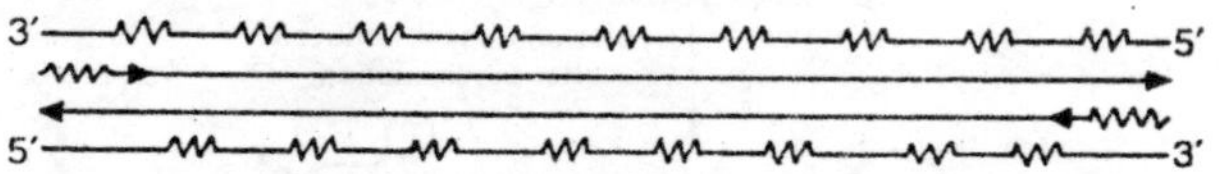

(b) 'gene amplification' using primers complementary to 3′ ends (∿∿ = gap filled by PCR)

Synthesis of gene using polymerase chain reaction.

Crude synthetic oligonucleotides, synthesised on automatic synthesisers, were sometimes also used for rapid generation of duplex DNA fragments. In all these procedures oligos are first phosphorylated at the 5′ ends, overlapping ends annealed, gaps filled by enzymatic extension at the 3′ends and finally nicks were joined with DNA ligase. The full length double strand DNA could be cloned in a plasmid/phage vector and multiplied in *E. coli.* Alternatively, it could be amplified by PCR, separated on gel, purified from gel and cloned.

The above steps of phosphorylation, annealing, gap filling, ligation and cloning could be dispensed with, in some of the recent methods of gene synthesis. For instance, overlapping oligonucleotides could be extended through several rounds of PCR. Full length double stranded DNA could then be amplified using short primers complementary to the 5′ ends of two strands. Recently (reported in December, 1996) at Lucknow, Dr. Rakesh Tuli and his group standardised a method for construction of synthetic genes.

In this method, overlapping oligos (6-16 base) with gaps between adjacent oligos, belonging to the same strand, were first synthesised on an automatic DNA synthesiser; complementary oligos were annealed using 14-18 base long overlaps and the assembled double stranded DNA was used for PCR to give complete DNA sequence by several cycles of PCR (Fig.). Deep Vent polymerase, instead of Taq polymerase was used to reduce error rate.

Synthesis of gene from mRNA H. Temin and D. Baltimore, in 1970 discovered the presence of 'RNA directed DNA polymerase' enzyme which has the ability of synthesizing DNA on RNA template. This enabled molecular biologists to synthesise complementary DNA (cDNA) using mRNA as a template. If mRNA transcribed from a specific gene is made available in purified form, the complementary DNA (cDNA) synthesised with its help will represent the synthesised gene. To what extent this synthesised gene is a faithful copy of native gene will depend on the fidelity of copying mRNA and also on the stability of cDNA thus synthesised. Moreover, since mRNA of a gene does not have the complete transcript of the gene *in vivo*, the synthesised gene will be smaller than the gene *in vivo*.

By copying eukaryotic purified mRNA, several genes have been artificially synthesised. Most important of these genes are the genes for sea urchin histone proteins, ovalbumin gene in chicken and globin genes in mammals.

The gene synthesised as cDNA from a (β globin mRNA, has been inserted into a plasmid in order to study its behaviour. As earlier pointed out, these genes will lack any additional regulatory sequences absent in mRNA but present in a globin gene *in vivo*. This type of gene will also lack intron sequences found in eukaryotic split genes. These genes (cDNA), however, have already become a very important tool in molecular biology experiments.

3

Role of Micromolecules

Cells of all living organisms are made up of chemicals, which obey the laws of chemistry and physics. Therefore, in this chapter, we briefly discuss the chemistry of the cell. In this chapter we describe micromolecules or small molecules, which are the basic ingredients of the cell.

The most abundant component of a living cell is water, making about 70% of cell's mass. However, if we disregard water, most micromolecules in a cell are carbon compounds involving other elements like hydrogen, nitrogen and oxygen. The simple rules of covalent bonding between carbon and other elements permit an infinitely large number of compounds, in which groups like methyl ($-CH_3$), hydroxyl (-OH), carboxyl (-COOH) and amino ($-NH_2$) occur repeatedly in living systems.

Thousands of different micromolecules present in the cell make only a small fraction of the total organic matter in a cell (Table). They can be broadly classified into: (i) simple sugars, (ii) fatty acids, (iii) amino acids, (iv) nucleotides and (v) lipids. These micro-molecules will be described in this chapter.

The Approximate Chemical Composition of a Bacterial Cell (modified from Alberts et. al., 1994)

Chemical constituent	Proportion (% total weight)	Number of types of each molecule
1. Water	70.0	1
2. Inorganic ions	1.0	20
3. Sugars and precursors	1.0	250
4. Amino acids and precursors	0.4	100
5. Nucleotides and precursors	0.4	100
6. Fatty acids and precursors	1.0	50
7. Other small molecules	0.2	300
8. Macromolecules	26.0	3000

Sugars (Carbohydrates)

Sugars or carbohydrates are usually classified into three groups: (i) monosaccharides, (ii) oligosaccharides and (iii) polysaccharides. Simplest sugars are monosaccharides with the general formula $(CH_5O)_n$, where n is an integer ranging

Common Monosacharides

Monosachardes With general formula (CH_2O).	Examples	
	Aldehydes	Ketones
1 Trioses, $C_3H_6O_3$	Glyceraldehyde	Dihydroxyacetone
2 Tetroses, $C_4H_8O_4$	Erythrose	Erythrulose
3 Pentoses, $C_5H_{10}O_5$	Deoxyribose	Ribose
4 Hexoses, $C_6H_{12}O_S$	Glucose	Fructose

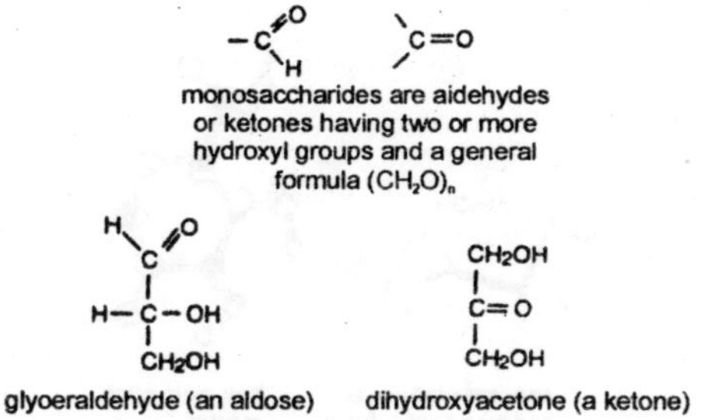

Two simplest monosaccharides, glyceraldehyde and dihydroxyacetone.

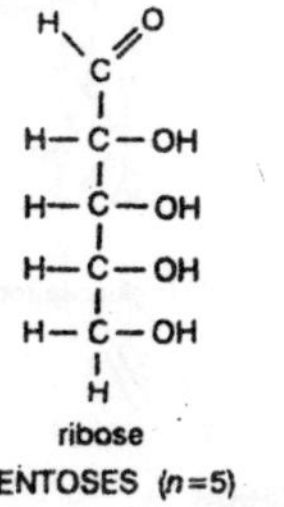

A common pentose-ribose sugar.

from 3 to 7. The simplest of these monosaccharides are those, with n = 3 giving a molecular formula $C_3H_6O_3$ represented by compounds like glyceraldehyde (an aldehyde) or dihydroxyacetone (a ketone) shown in Figure (Table). Another class of common monosaccharides is represented by pentoses (ribose and deoxyribose), which are used as building blocks for nucleotides and nucleic acids (Fig.). However, the most common monosaccharide found in the cell is glucose with the formula $C_6H_{12}O_6$ and having either an open chain form or a

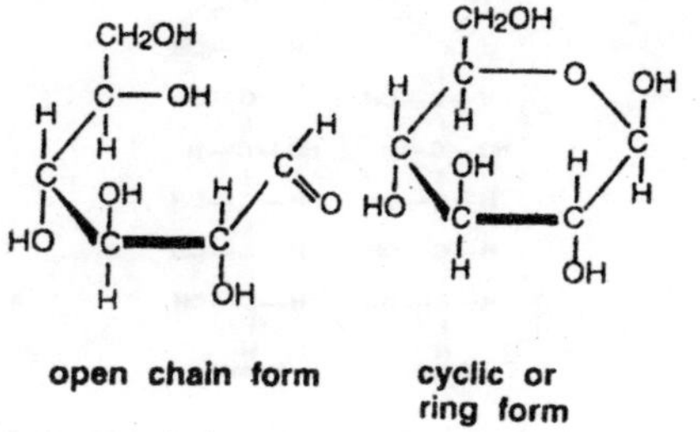

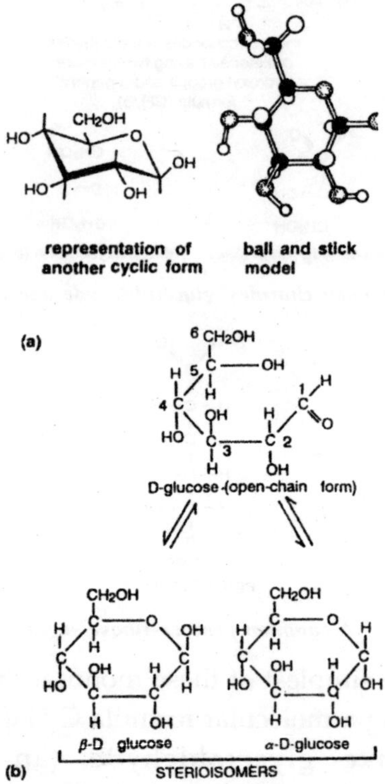

(a) Open and closed-chain forms of glucose (a common hexose sugar); (b) two stereoisomers of glucose (β-D-glucose and α-D-glucose). are in balance with open form.

ring form (Fig.). In their open chain form, in addition to a number of hydroxyl groups, sugars contain either an aldehyde

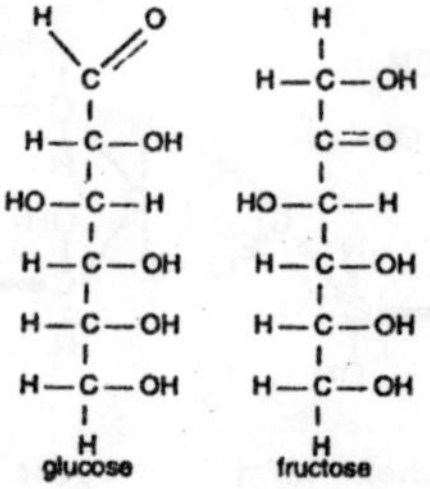

Two common haxoses-glucose and fructose.

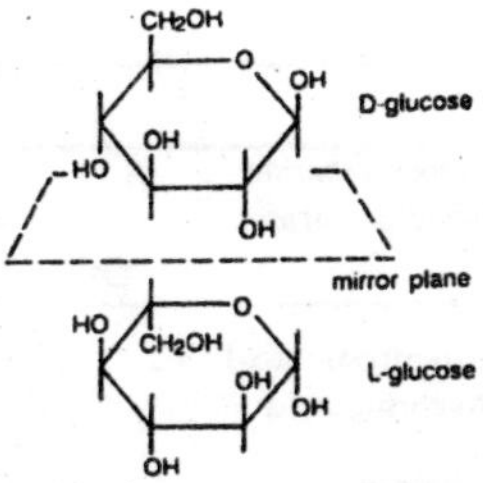

D-glucose and L-glucose are mirror image of each other.

(H - C = O) group as in glucose or a keto (C=O) group as in fructose (Fig.). The aldehyde or keto group can react with a hydroxyl group in the same molecule to convert open chain into a ring form, which can exist in several isomeric forms (*e.g.*, D-glucose and L-glucose; α -D glucose and β -D glucose; see Fig.). In its ring form, the carbon of the original aldehyde or keto group can be recognised as the only carbon atom, that is bonded with two oxygens. The hydroxyl groups of a simple monosaccharide can also be replaced by other groups to give derived monosaccharides (Table). Further, in its ring form, the carbon of the original aldehyde or ketone group in a sugar molecule can become linked to another sugar molecule (through one of its carbon atoms bearing a hydroxyl group) to form a disaccharide. This phenomenon is described as condensation (the reverse process being hydrolysis). The linkage between two monosaccharide sugar molecules is called glycosidic linkage

Derived Monosaccharides.

Class of derived monosaccharide	*Examples*	
	Monosaccharide	*Corresponding derived monosaccharide*
1. Glycoside Galactose	Glucose Galactosides	Glucoside
2. Sugar phosphates	Glucose	Glucose-1 phosphate
	Glucose	Glucose-6-phosphate
3. Sugar acids (C-l oxidised to -COOH)	Glucose	Gluconic acid

Contd...

Class of derived	Examples	
	Monosaccharide monosaccharide	*Corresponding derived monosaccharide*
Glucose Vitamin C	Glucuronic acid Ascorbic acid	(C-6 oxidised to -COOH)
4. Amino sugars (hexosamines) Galactose	Glucose ? ? ?	Glucosamine, N-acetyl glucosamine N-acetylgalactosamine N-acetyl muramic acid, Neuraminic acid, Sialic acid

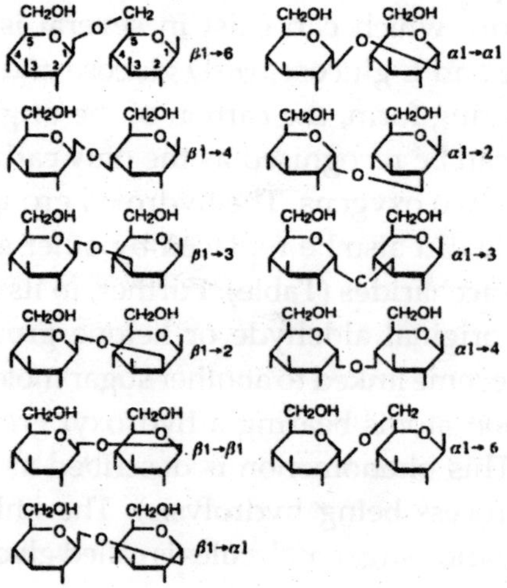

Eleven disaccharides, each consisting of two D-glucose units, and differing only in the type of linkage (shown against each molecule).

Details of Constitution of Some Disaccharides

Dissacharide constituents	*Monosaccharide Linkage*	*Glycosidic*
1. Lactose D-galactose	D-glucose +	β-1,4
2. Maltose D-glucose	D-glucose +	α-1,4

Contd....

	Dissacharide constituents	*Monosaccharide Linkage*	*Glycosidic*
3.	Cellobiose D-glucose	D-glucose +	β -1,4
4.	Isomaltose D-glucose	D-glucose +	α -1,4
5.	Sucrose D-fructose	D-glucose +	α -1, - β 2

or glycosidic bond, because the hydroxyl group at carbon atom no. 1 (C-l), which is involved in this linkage is described as glycosidic hydroxyl. Depending upon the positions of carbon atoms in two monosaccharide molecules involved in glycosidic linkage, the linkage can be described as 1-4, 1-6 or 1-2. Further, depending upon the a or (3 forms of each of the two molecules (or α form of one molecule and β form of the other molecule) involved in linkage, the linkages can be described as follows: α -1, 4 linkage; β -l, 4 linkage; α -1, 6 linkage and α -1, β -2 linkage, etc. Even a simple disaccharide consisting of two glucose residues can exist in eleven different forms (Fig.). Some of the common disaccharides, their monosaccharide constituents and glycosidic linkages are summarised in Table.

Several trisaccharides ($C_{18}H_{36}O_{18}$) of biological importance are also known. Raffinose is one such trisaccharide with monosaccharide units, D-glucose, D-fructose and D-galactose. Other trisaccharides are mannotriose, rabinose, rhamminose, gentianose and melezitose. Sugars of higher order are also known. The sugars consisting of fewer sugar residues (generally 2-9) are often collectively described as oligosaccharides.

Sugars having a large number of monosaccharide units (often having atleast 10 units) are known as polysaccharides These are classified according to their monosaccharide units, *e.g.*, glucans consisting of glucose monomers and galactans consisting of galactose monomers. These polysaccharides represent a class of macromolecules.

Acids regarding Fats

A fatty acid molecule has two distinct regions: (i) a long hydrocarbon chain, *e.g.*, $CH_3\ (CH_2)_n$ which is hydrophobic (water insoluble) and chemically not very reactive, and (ii) a carboxylic group (-COOH), which ionises in solution giving COO^-, thus being hydrophilic (water soluble) and chemically reactive. The carboxylic group reacts with a hydroxyl or an amino group of a second molecule to form esters (lipids) or amides respectively.

All fatty acid molecules in a cell are usually covalently linked to other molecules by their carboxylic acid group. Hundreds of different kinds of fatty acids exist in the cells and differ firstly in the length of the hydrocarbon chain and secondly in being either saturated having no double bonds (*e.g.*, palmitic acid), or unsaturated having one double bond (monoenoic acids, *e.g.*, oleic acid), two double bonds (dienoic acids, *e.g.*, linoleic acid), three double bonds (trienoic acids, *e.g.*, linolenic acid) or even many double bonds (polyenoic acids, *e.g.*, arachidonic acid) (Table).

Some Unsaturated Fatty Acids

Class of unsaturated fatty acid	Fatty acid	Chemical formula showing double bonds
Monoenoic	Oleic acid	$CH_3(CH_2)_7CH = CH(CH_2)_7COOH$
Dienoic	Linoleic acid	$CH_3(CH_2)_4CH = CH - CH_2 - CH = CH(CH_2)_7COOH$
Trienoic	Linolenic acid	$CH_3 - CH_2 - CH = CH - CH_2 - CH = CH - CH_2 - CH = CH(CH_2)_7COOH$
Tetraenoic	Arachidonic acid	$CH_3(CH_2)_4CH = CH.CH_2.CH = CHCH_2CH = CHCH_2CH = CH(CH_2)_3COOH$

As components of lipids, fatty acids are a valuable source of food, since they can be broken down to produce more than twice as much usable energy as glucose (weight by weight). Fatty acids, In the form of droplets of triglyceride molecules are stored in the cytoplasm of many cells and represent animal fats. When required, fatty acids are released from these triglycerides and are broken down into two-carbon units to release energy. These two-carbon units, present in the form of acetyl coenzyme A (acetyl CoA), are further degraded in various energy yielding reactions.

Fatty acids are also found as phospholipids and glycolipids forming an important component of cell membranes (see later for structure of phospholipids).

Amino Acids: All amino acids contain a carboxylic group and an amino group, both linked to a single carbon atom called the α -carbon (Fig.). They are the building blocks of proteins, which are a class of macromolecules consisting of amino acids joined by peptide bonds. A peptide bond is formed between the carboxylic group of one amino acid and the amino group of the adjoining amino acid (Fig.).

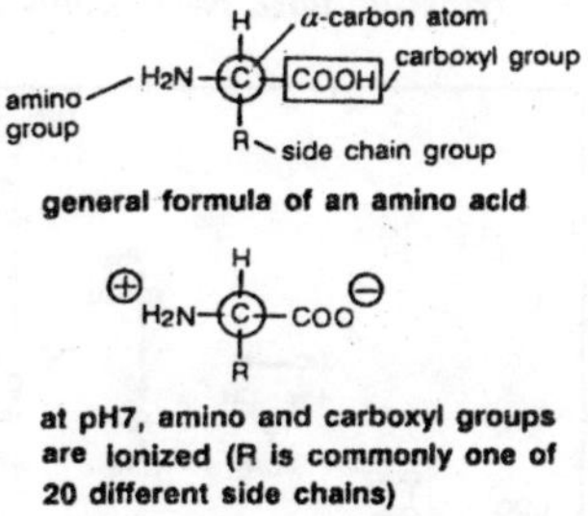

The general formula of an amino acid showing the positions of amino (-NH$_2$) group, carboxyl group (-COOH), α *-carbon atom and a side chain.*

Although, there can be many different kinds of amino acids, their number approaching 100, only 20 of them are commonly found in proteins in all classes of organisms ranging from bacteria to higher plants and animals. Different amino acids have an -NH$_2$ group, a -COOH group and an α -carbon in common, but differ with respect to the structure of side chain attached to the α -carbon. These 20 amino acids occurring in proteins are so selected during evolution, that they provide considerable chemical versatility. Five (aspartic acid, glutamic acid, histidine, lysine, arginine) of these 20 amino acids carry each a side chain that can carry a charge, but other 15 are

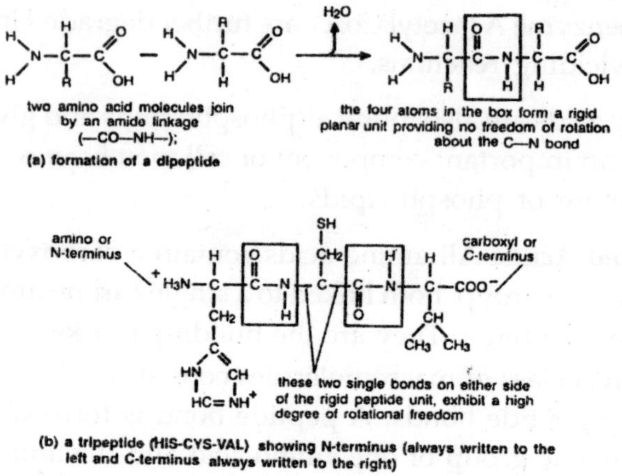

(a) Formation of a peptide bond between two amino acids giving a dipeptide and (b) a tripetide with N-terminus and C-terminus.

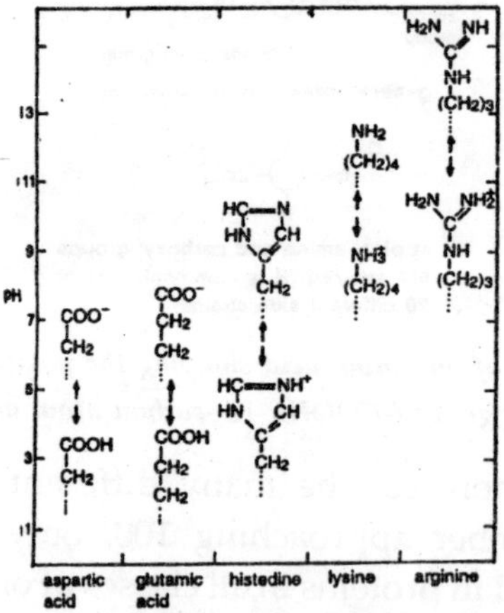

The dependence of the charge on the side chain of an amino acid on the pH; the carboxylic group of the acid loses H⁺ in aqueous solution and degree of this dissociation depends on pH thus controlling the charge; the pH at which exactly half of the carboxylic acid is charged in an amino acid, is known as its pK (redrawn from Alberts et. al.: Molecular Biology of the Cell, 1994).

uncharged, though reactive in various specific ways. The charge on the amino acids depends on pH of the solution. In aqueous solution, each of the above five amino acids lose H^+ to form a negatively charged ion (*e.g.* aspartate, glutamate, etc.). In this respect amines are comparable and become positively charged by accepting a H^+. In a solution, both charged and uncharged forms of an amino acid may be found, their relative proportion depending on the pH of the solution. For instance, at high pH, an amino acid is charged and an amine is uncharged and at low pH the situation is reverse. The pH at which half of the carboxylic acid or amine residues are charged is known as the pK of that amino acid side chain (Fig.). In the cell, pH is close to 7 so that all carboxylic acid and amine residues are in their fully charged form.

The amino acids are grouped according to whether their side chains are: (i) acidic, (ii) basic, (iii) uncharged polar and (iv) nonpolar (Fig). Amino acids with acidic or basic side chains are very polar and are always found on the outside of protein molecules. The amino acids with uncharged polar side chains are hydrophilic and they are also found on the outside of proteins, but those with non-polar side chains are found inside the protein molecules. Paired cysteines also allow formation of disulphide bonds during formation of proteins. The properties and functions of proteins actually depend on the properties of amino acid side chains found in their constituent amino acids.

Abbreviations for 20 Essential Amino Acids

Amino acid	*Abbreviations*	
	Three letter	*One letter*
Alanine	Ala	A
Cysteine	Cys	C
Aspartic acid	Asp	D
Glutamic acid	Glu	E

Contd...

Amino acid	*Abbreviations*	
	Three letter	*One letter*
Phenylalanine*	Phe	F
Glycine	Gly	G
Histidine*	His	H
Isoleucine*	lie	I
Lysine*	Lys	K
Leucine*	Leu	L
Methionine*	Met	M
Asparagine	Asn	N
Proline	Pro	P
Glutamine	Gin	Q
Arginine	Arg	R
Serine	Ser	S
Threonine*	Thr	T
Valine*	Val	V
Tryptophan*	Trp	W
Tyrosine	Tyr	Y

(nine essential amino acids are each matted with an asterisk)

The 20 amino acids found in proteins have been each given both a three letter and one letter abbreviations. Of these 20 amino acids, nine are essential amino acids (Table).

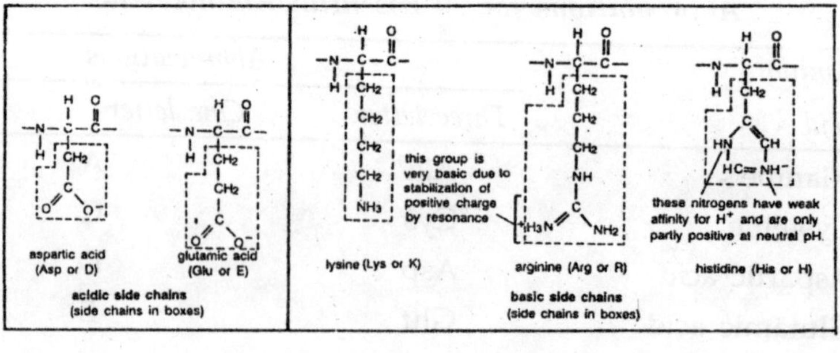

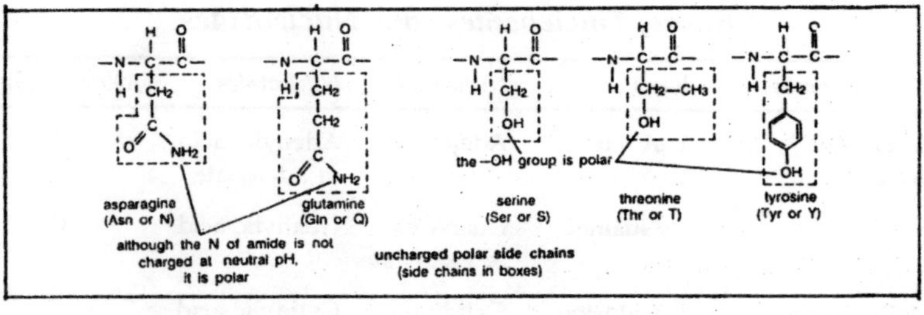

Four families of amino acids, grouped according to acidic and basic nature of the side chain and the charge carried by this side chain.

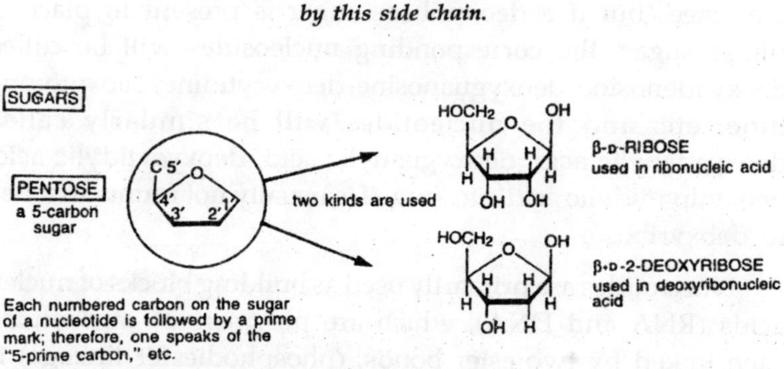

Two pentose sugars, β-D-ribose found in RNA and β-D-2-deoxyribose found in DNA.

Bases, Nucleosides and Nucleotides

Class of Bases	*Bases*	*Nucleosides*	*Nucleotides*	*Abbreviations*
I. Purine bases	1. Adenine	Adenosine	Adenylic acid or adenylate	A
	2. Guanine	Guanosine or guanylate	Guanylic acid	G
II. Pyrimidine bases	1. Cytosine	Cytidine	Cytidylic acid or cytidylate	C
	2. Uracil	Uridine or uridylate	Uridylic acid	U
	3. Thymine	Thymidine or thymidylate	Thymidylic acid	T

The Nucleotides

A nucleotide consists of a nucleoside, to which a phosphate group is attached, and a nucleoside in its turn consists of a base (so called because it can combine with H^+ in acidic solution) linked to a five-carbon sugar (also called pentose), which may be ribose or deoxyribose (Fig.). The nucleosides or nucleotides can be of five types and their names are derived from the bases they contain (Table). In Table the nomenclature of only ribonucleosides and ribonucleotides having ribose sugar residue are listed, but if a deoxyribose sugar is present in place of ribose sugar, the corresponding nucleosides will be called deoxyadenosine, deoxyguanosine, deoxycytidine, deoxythymidine, etc. and the nucleotides will be similarly called deoxyadenylic acid, deoxyguanylic acid, deoxycytidylic acid, deoxythymidylic acid, etc. (uracil is usually not found attached to deoxyribose).

Nucleotides are primarily used as building blocks of nucleic acids (RNA and DNA), which are polymers of nucleotides, each linked by two ester bonds, (phosphodiester linkage) to another nucleotide (Fig.). There are two main types of nucleic acids, which differ in the type of sugar, which forms the backbone: (i) ribose sugar is found in ribonucleic acid or RNA, which contains the bases A,U,G and C and (ii) deoxyribose sugar (where oxygen at position 2 is missing) is found in DNA. The sequence of bases in DNA or RNA represents the genetic information.

Nucleotides have many functions other than the storage of genetic information. These functions include the following: (i) They carry chemical energy in their easily hydrolysed acid-anhydride bonds as in adenosine tri-phosphate or ATP (Fig.). The triphosphate ester of ATP participates in the transfer of energy in hundreds of individual cellular reactions. The terminal phosphate during the production of ATP is added using energy

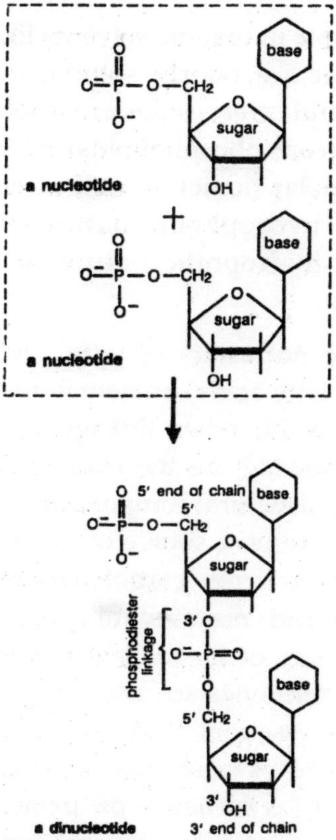

Two nucleotides joining by a phosphodiester bond to form a dinucleotide.

from oxidation of food stuffs and this phosphate can be split off readily by hydrolysis to release energy for other reactions within the cell, (ii) Nucleotides also combine with other groups to form enzymes as in coenzyme A or CoA (see Fig.). (iii) Nucleotides like cyclic adenosine monophosphate (cyclic AMP or cAMP) are also used as specific signaling molecules in the cell (Fig.).

Lipids: Lipids are naturally occurring biomolecules comprising a large and diverse group of compounds that are saponifiable esters of long chain (saturated or unsaturated) fatty acids.

They are soluble in organic solvents like chloroform, ether and benzene, but are poorly soluble in water. However, sphingomyelins and cerebrosides are insoluble in ether, while phosphatides (glycero-phospholipids) are insoluble in acetone. The lipids have polar (ionic) as well as nonpolar (nonrionic) groups, so that hydrophobic nature of hydrocarbons is associated with hydrophilic nature of other groups like carboxylic group.

All lipids are not esters of fatty acids. For instance, in cerebrosides, the fatty acids's moiety is an amide and in many other lipids there are ether linkages (*e.g.*, ether lipids or plasmogens). Following are the main biological functions of lipids: (i) they are structural components- of all living systems; (ii) they are major reserve source of energy, giving 9.7kcal/g, twice that obtained from carbohydrates -this is used for muscular work and maintenance of body temperature; (iii) they are carriers of fat-soluble vitamins A, D, E and K; (iv) some of the hormones are also lipids or their derivatives; (v) they provide essential fatty acids such as linoleic and linolenic acids; some of these fatty acids (*e.g.*, linoleic acid) are precursors for biosynthesis of prostaglandins, which are essential for maintaining several functions of the body (see later in this chapter).

Lipids can be either simple lipids which yield monohydric or trihydric alcohol and fatty acid on hydrolysis (due to lipases) or they may be complex lipids, which contain phosphate, various sugars and nitrogenous compounds such as sphingosine, ethanolamine and serine. A summary of the classification of lipids is presented in Figure.

Fats and Waxes

Fats and waxes are esters of fatty acids with alcohols; while fats are esters of fatty acids with glycerol (*e.g.*, triglycerides), waxes are esters of fatty acids with higher chain length aliphatic

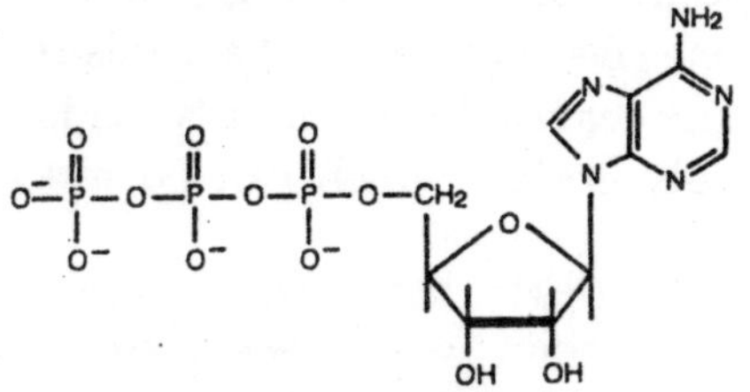

they carry chemical energy in their easily hydrolysed acid- anhydride bonds (e.g. ATP)

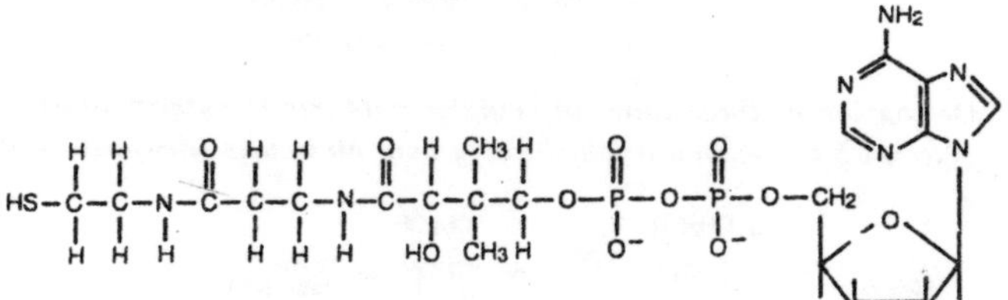

they combine with other groups to form enzymes (e.g. coenzyme A or CoA)

they are used as specific signaling molecules in the cell (e.g. cyclic AMP or cAMP)

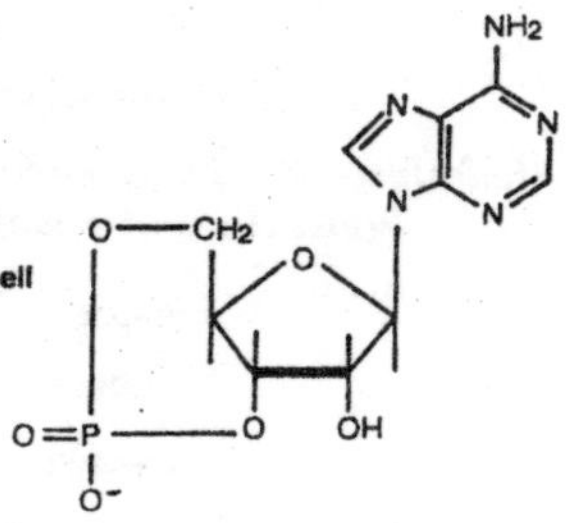

Three nucleotides, which are not parts of nucleic acids, and have functions other than storage of genetic information.

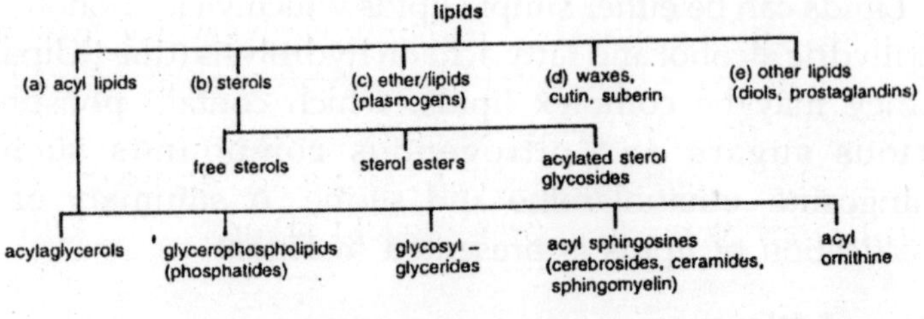

A classification of lipids, showing five main groups and their further division into sub-groups.

monohydric alcohols (*e.g.*, lanonin, secreted in the skin of most fur bearing animals; spermaceti, a wax found in the sperm whale as a source of stored energy, and myricyl palmitate secreted by honey bee = Bee wax). Waxes also serve as protective coatings on fruit leaves. Esters of fatty acids with glycerol are described as glycerides, which can be monoglycerides, *i.e.*,

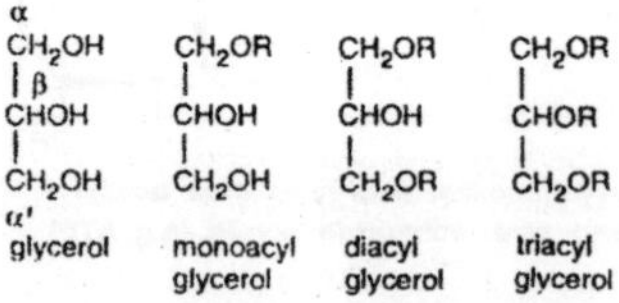

R = fatty acid residue = $-OCO(CH_2)_n CH_3$

Derivation of three types of acylglycerols due to esterification of glycerol by one, two or three fatty acid molecules (denoted as R)

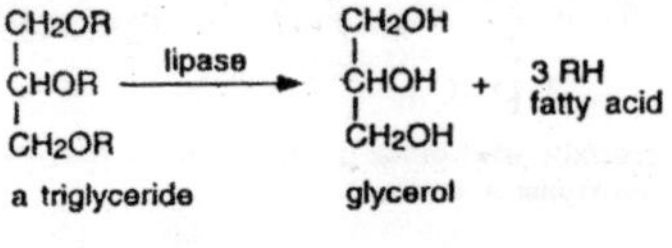

$R = CH_3(CH_2)_n COO^-$

Hydrolysis of a triglyceride to yield three fatty acid molecules and a molecule of glycerol.

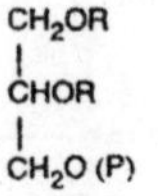

3sn-phosphatidic acid

A phosphatidic acid molecule, which is glycerophosphoric acid esterified with two molecules of fatty acid.

monoacyl glycerol (when one hydroxyl group of glycerol is esterified) or diglycerides, *i.e.*, diacyl glycerol (when two hydroxyl groups of glycerol are esterified) or triglycerides, *i.e.*, triacyl glycerol (when all the three hydroxyl groups are esterified; see Fig.).

Monoglycerides and diglycerides are not so common and are actually intermediates in biosynthesis of triglycerides, which are the common neutral fats, found as main energy storing compounds in the body. A triglyceride on hydrolysis with the help of lipases yields fatty acids and glycerol (Fig.). When molecules of the same fatty acid are involved at all the three ester bonds, triglyceride is described as simple, but when they differ, the triglyceride is described as mixed.

Glycerophospholipids (Phosphatides)

Glycerophospholipids or phosphatides, as the word indicates, are phospholipids (an alcohol + fatty acid + phosphoric acid), which are derivatives of glycerophosphatidic acid (glycerol having two fatty acid groups and a phosphoric acid group; see Fig). These are widely distributed in animal and plant tissues.

The phosphatides differ in the nature of their fatty acids and in the nature of the alcohol (*e.g.*, aminoalcohols, inositols), which is esterified to phosphoric acid group of phosphatidic acid. Four of these phosphatides are shown in Figure. Of these phosphatides, lecithins are the most abundant and phosphatidyl inositols are frequently used in signal transduction pathways.

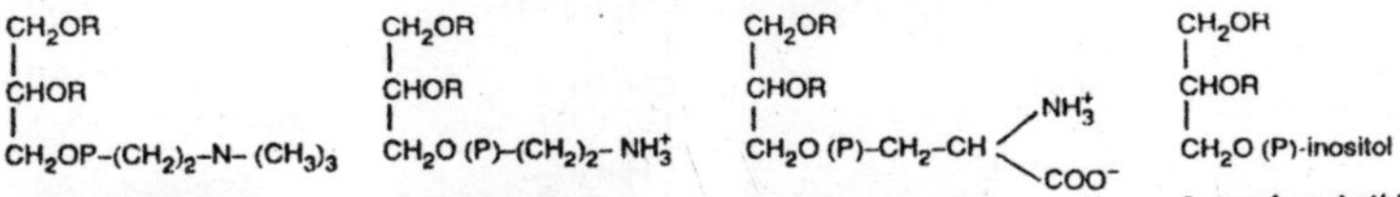

3 sn–phosphatidyl choline (lecithin) — 3 sn–phosphatidyl ethanolamine — 3 sn–phosphatidyl serine — 3 sn–phosphatidyl inositol

Four different phosphatides derived due to esterification of the phosphoric acid group of the phosphatidic acid, by different groups (choline, ethanolamine, serine, inositol).

Glycoglycerides

Glycoglycerides are lipids with a carbohydrate moiety attached to sn-3 position of glycerol and are mainly found in photosynthetic membranes of higher plants and cyanobacteria. In small quantities they are also found in fungi and bacteria. Common examples are diacylgalactosyl glycerol and diacyl digalactosyl glycerol (Fig.).

Acyl Sphingosines, Sphingoglycolipids and Sphingophospholipids

Acyl sphingosines and sphingophospholipids are fatty acid derivatives of sphingosine (Fig.), and are widely distributed in plants and animals respectively. Fatty acid residues are usually saturated and each contains a long carbon chain (*e.g.*, lignoceric acid). They include ceramides (acyl sphingosines) cerebroside (ceramides with carbohydrate group; sphingoglycolipids) and sphingomyelines (sphingophospholipids).

diacylgalactosyl glycerol   diacyldigalactosyl glycerol

Diacylgalactosyl glycerol and diacyldigalactosyl glycerol where two hydroxyl groups of glycerol condense with acyl groups and the third is condensed with one or two galactose molecules.

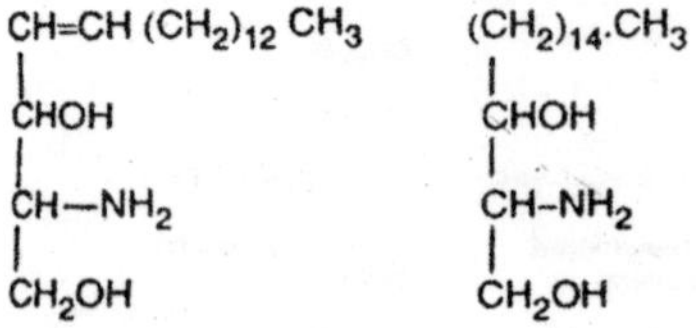

sphingosine   **dihydroxy-sphingosine**

A sphingosine molecule, and a dihydroxysphingosine molecule.

Steroids and Sterols: Unlike true lipids and phospholipids, steroids and sterols do not contain fatty acids. In animals, steroids include cholesterol, hormone secreted by testis, ovary and adrenal cortex (except relaxin Table), vitamin D precursors,

Hormones Secreted by Testis, Ovary and Adrenal Cortex, with their Characteristics

Hormones	*Number of C atoms*	*Structure*
1. Male hormones		No side chain at
(a) testosterone	19	C–17; oxo –or
(b) androsterone		hydroxy groups at C–3 and C–17
2. Female hormones		
(a) oestrogens (oesterone)	18	A benzenoid ring; hydroxyl group at C–3
(b) progesterone	21	A two-carbon side chain at C–17
3. Adrenal cortex hormones		
(a) glucocorticoids (*e.g.*, cortisol)	21	A two-carbon side chain at C–17;
(b) oxo-or mineralo-corticoids (*e.g.*, 11–dexycortisol)		oxo/hydroxy groups at C–3, C–ll, C–17

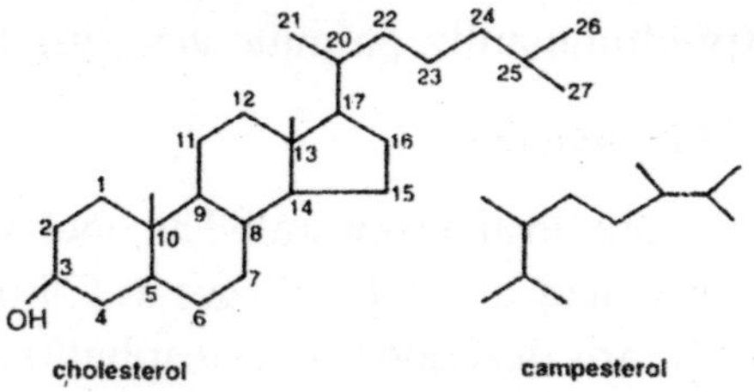

Structure of a cholesterol molecule and a campesterol molecule.

bile acids (catabolic products of cholesterol) and bile salts. In plants, sterols are found either in free form or as sterol esters, acylated sterol glycosides or sterol-glycosides.

Steroids are derived from squalene, a 30-carbon compound, and contain a nucleus (called cyclopentano perhydrophenanthrene nucleus) consisting of three 6-membered carbon rings (A,B and C) and one 5-membered ring (D), with all the rings fully saturated. The carbon atoms of the nucleus are numbered 1 to 17. Sterols are steroids with a hydroxyl group at carbon 3, and a carbon 17 side chain containing about 10 carbon atoms (*e.g.*, cholesterol; Fig.).

Cholesterol is found in cell membranes (of many organisms), blood and bile. It is also a precursor of several hormones including cortisones testosterone, estrogen, progesterone and other steroid hormones. Ergosterol is precursor of vitamin D.

Free sterols found in plants include sitosterol, stigmasterol and campesterol, which differ in degree of substitution and unsaturation.

Sterol esters are also found in plants and involve esterification of the 3-OH group with a fatty acid (*e.g.*, palmitoyl sterol). Acylated sterol glycosides are storage compounds for sterol and represent its transportable form; they are sterol derivatives, where 3-OH group forms a glycosidic linkage with sugar (usually glucose) and 6th position is esterified with a fatty acid (predominantly palmitic acid/linoleic acid).

Ether Lipids (Plasmogens)

These lipids contain an unsaturated alcohol in ether linkage (instead of a fatty acid in ester linkage) at C-l of L-glycero-3-phosphate. They are described as phosphatidal, rather than phosphatides (see earlier). Some of the ether lipids called plasmogens, contain at their phosphate end, an ethanolamine (phosphatidal etnanolamine), choline (phosphatidal choline) or serine (phosphatidal serine). They are mainly found in fungi, anaerobic bacteria and higher plants.

Prostaglandins

They are cyclopentoic acids, which are cyclic and hydroxylated derivatives of polyunsaturated fatty acids like arachidonic acid. The different prostaglandins (*e.g.*, PG_E, PG_F and PG_H) differ from each other in the substituted cyclopentane ring and R_1 and R_2 groups (Fig) prostaglandins were first discovered in human seminal fluid (hence this name), testis, placenta, uterus, stomach, lung, brain and heart.

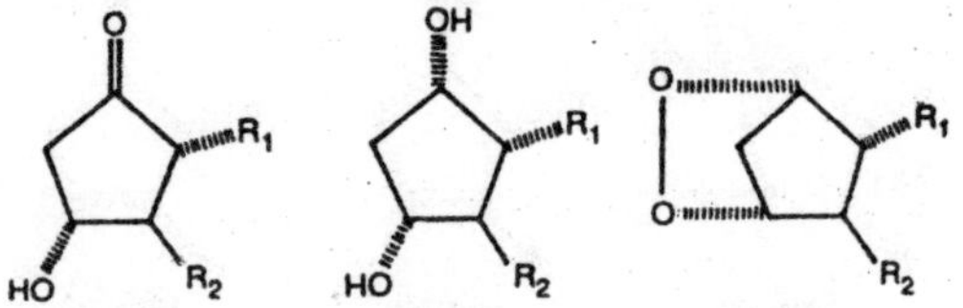

(a) PG_E (b) PG_F (c) PG_H

Three different proslaglandins.

4

Process of Metabolism

As a result of digestion, proteins are broken down into *amino acids,* carbohydrates into simple sugars (mainly *glucose)* and fats into *fatty acids and glycerol.* In the intestine the amino acids and sugars are absorbed into the blood vessels, and fatty acids and glycerol into lymphatic vessels, from where they are carried to the tissues. Within the cells, the molecules are metabolised to provide energy, or are built up into other molecules. This process is called *intermediary metabolism.* Metabolism consists of two processes, *catabolism* and *anabolism.* In *catabolism,* degradation of complex organic molecules into simpler molecules takes place, usually by *oxidative reactions.* In this process energy is released. *Anabolism* is the process of biosynthesis in which complex molecules are produced from simpler molecules. This is usually done by *reduction reactions,* and energy is required for the process.

Metabolism of Carbohydrate

Sixty per cent of injested food consists of *polysaccharide carbohydrates. Disaccharide* carbohydrates like *sucrose* are also of some importance, while *lactose* or milk sugar is important in the diet of infants. The end product of carbohydrate digestion is mainly glucose. Some *fructose* and *galactose* may also be formed. These simple sugars are absorbed in the intestine and are carried to the liver through the blood stream. Here they are transformed into *glycogen* through *glucose 6-phosphate.* Glycogen is stored in the liver. When glucose is required, the glycogen breaks down into glucose, which is then utilised as a source of energy by the cells of the body. The greatest amount is used by muscle cells, and a considerable amount by nerve cells. Other tissues use lesser amounts.

Respiration in Cell

During cell respiration food materials are oxidised to carbon dioxide and water in the presence of oxygen. One of the most important fuels is glucose. The overall equation for cell respiration in the presence of oxygen is:

$$C_6H_{12}O_6 + 6O_2 \rightarrow 6CO_2 + 6H_2O + \text{Energy}$$

Under aerobic conditions glucose metabolism takes place in four stages, glycolysis, pyruvic acid oxidation, Krebs citric acid cycle and oxidative phosphorylation in the hydrogen/electron transfer system (Fig.).

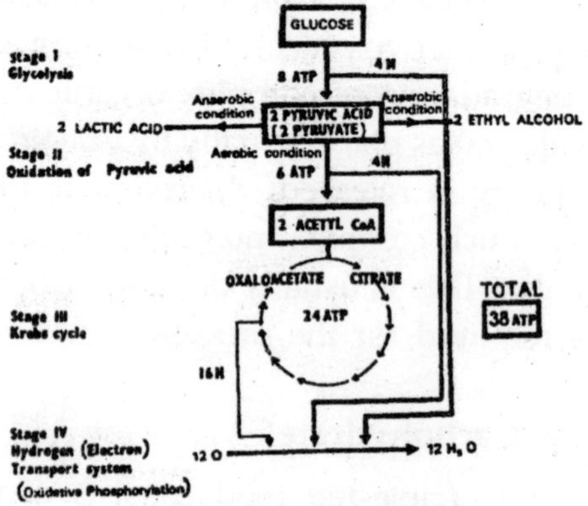

Outline of cell respiration.

Glycolysis: The breakdown of glucose to pyruvic acid is called glycolysis. Glycolysis can take place in the absence of oxygen (*anaerobic* condition) or in the presence of oxygen (*aerobic* condition). The enzymes for glycolysis are found in the soluble fraction of the cell, out side the mitochondria.

Pyruvic Acid Oxidation: Under aerobic conditions the pyruvic acid molecule is metabolised to a molecule of *acetyl coenzyme A* (acetyl CoA).

Krebs Citric Acid Cycle: Each acetyl CoA molecule condenses with a molecule of oxaloacetic acid to produce a molecule of *citric acid.* After several steps oxaloacetic acid is regenerated. Krebs cycle takes place under aerobic conditions. The enzymes for the Krebs cycle are located in the matrix of the mitochondrion.

Oxidative Phosphorylation in the Hydrogen Transfer System: Several pairs of hydrogen atoms are released during glycolysis, pyruvic acid oxidation and the Krebs cycle. These are passed through the election transfer system, and are finally accepted by molecular oxygen.

During this process ADP is phosphorylated to ATP with inorganic phosphate. The enzymes of the hydrogen transport system are located in the inner membrane of the mitochondrion.

Stage I: Glycolysis

Glycolysis is the breakdown of glucose upto the formation of pyruvic acid. Other substances like glycogen and fructose may also be the starting compounds in glycolysis. The most common pathway in glycolysis is the *Embden-Meyerhof-Parnas* (EMP scheme) (Fig.). Among the other pathways are the *Entner-Duodoroff* scheme (ED scheme) and the *Hexose Monophosphate* scheme (HMP scheme). As mentioned previously, glycolysis can take place both in the absence of oxygen (*anaerobic* condition) or in the presence of oxygen (*aerobic* condition).

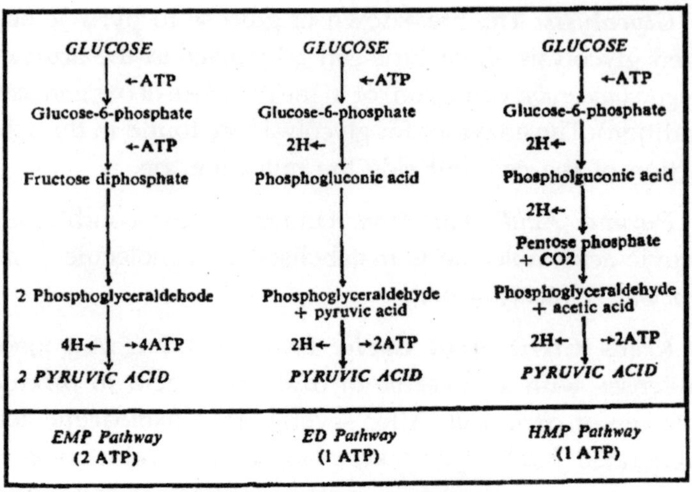

Some of the pathways of glycolysis.

Fate of Pyruvic Acid: The fate of pyruvic differs in the different types of respiration (Fig.).

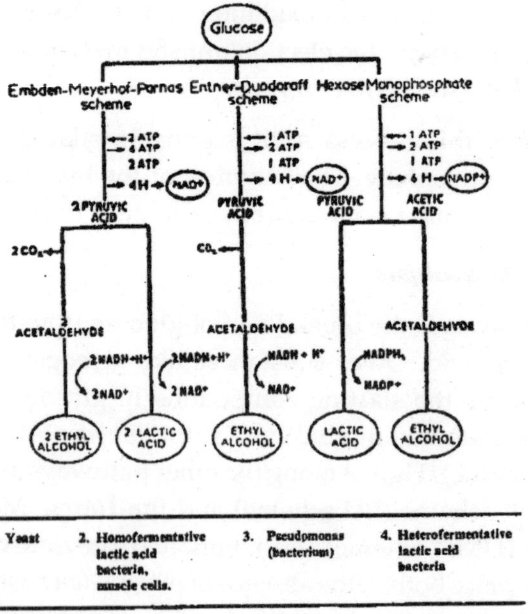

The fate of pyruvic acid in some of the pathways of glucose metabolism.

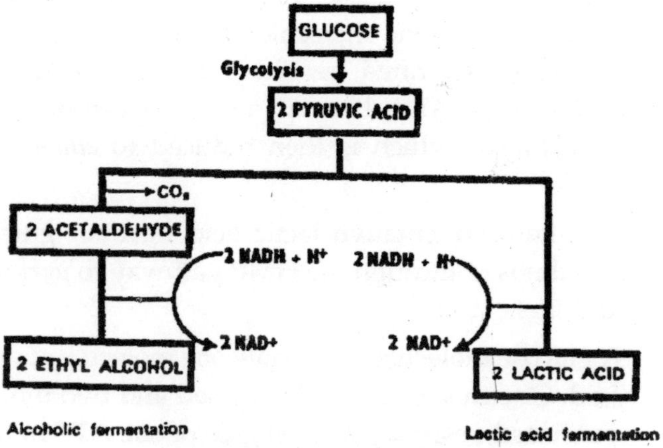

Alcoholic and lactic acid fermentation.

1. In yeast (*Saccharomyces* species) glucose is metabolised to pyruvic acid through the EMP pathway. Each glucose molecule yields two molecules of pyruvic acid. During glycolysis, two molecules of ATP are used and four are generated. Thus there is a net gain of two molecules of ATP per molecule of glucose metabolised. Pyruvic acid is decarboxylated to form *actaldehyde* and CO_2. Acetaldehyde serves as the final hydrogen acceptor. Reduction of acetaldehyde by $NADH_2$ produces *ethanol* (ethyl alcohol), and NAD^+ is regenerated.

2. Homolactic fermentation. In the lactic acid bacteria (e.g. *bacilli, lactobacilli, streptococci* and *clostridia)* a molecule of glucose yields two molecules of pyruvic acid through the EMP pathway. As in yeast, there is a net gain of two ATP molecules. Pyruvic acid itself is the final hydrogen acceptor. It is reduced by $NADH_2$ to yield lactic acid, and NAD^+ is regenerated. This type of fermentation is called *homolactic fermentation* because lactic acid is the sole product. The bacteria are called homofermentative lactic acid bacteria.

3. In the bacterium *Pseudomonas,* glucose gives rise to pyruvic acid through the ED pathway. In this bacterium

a molecule of glucose yields only one molecule of pyruvic acid. One molecule of ATP is used and two molecule generated, resulting in a net gain of one molecule of ATP. Pyruvic acid is decarboxylated to *acetaldehyde,* which is then reduced to *ethanol,* as in yeast.

4. In heterofermentative lactic acid bacteria glucose is metabolised through the HMP pathway to *pyruvic acid* and *acetic acid.*

   A glucose molecule yields only one molecule of pyruvic acid. One molecule of ATP is used and two molecules generated, resulting in a net gain of one ATP molecule. Pyruvic acid is reduced to *lactic acid,* and acetic acid to *acetaldehyde* and finally *ethanol.* The overall scheme is as follows:

   Glucose → Lactic acid + Ethanol + CO_2

5. In certain types of fermentation, e.g. alkaline fermentation in yeast, glucose yields glycerol as one of the products. There is no gain of ATP in this type of fermentation.

6. In most animal cells and aerobic micro-organisms pyruvic acid is oxidised to *acetyl CoA,* which then enters the Krebs cycle.

7. In skeletal muscle energy is required in sudden bursts. It is mostly released by glycolysis under relatively anaerobic conditions. When muscle contraction takes place under anaerobic conditions, pyruvic acid interacts with $NADH_2$ to yield *lactic acid,* and NAD^+ is regenerated.

   If contraction takes place under aerobic conditions then pyruvic acid is oxidised to CO_2 and H_2O through the Krebs citric acid cycle. In insect flight muscle lactic acid is not produced from glucose.

Glycolysis (Embden-Meyerhof-Parnas Scheme)

Glycolysis is the breakdown of glucose upto the formation of pyruvic acid (Fig.). Each glucose molecule forms two molecules of pyruvic acid. The breakdown takes place in a series of steps, each catalysed by a specific enzyme. At the end of the series the two pyruvic acid molecules retain most of the energy of the original glucose molecule. The reduction of glucose during glycolysis provides compounds for the synthesis of proteins, fats and nucleic acids. Most of the steps of glycolysis are reversible.

Glycolysis may be divided into two phases, a *preparatory* phase and an *oxidative* phase. In the following account glycolysis has been dealt with in 9 steps, of which steps 1 to 4 represent the preparatory phase and steps 5 to 9 the oxidative phase. In the preparatory phase breakdown of glucose and *low energy phosphorylation* occurs, and energy is *expended.* In the oxidative phase *high-energy* phosphate bonds are formed and energy is *stored.*

(1) Phosphorylation is the first step in the breakdown of carbohydrates. Glucose normally resists breakdown because it is a fairly stable compound. If its breakdown is to take place then it must first be made more reactive. The 'activation' of the glucose molecule takes place by a reaction called *oxidative phosphorylation.* A phosphate group is attached to glucose by a *low energy* phosphate bond (—P), and *glucose-6-phosphate* (activated glucose) is formed. The reaction is facilitated by the enzyme *hexokinase, with* Mg^{++} as an activator. The phosphate group is derived from ATP which breaks down to ADP. Starch or glycogen may also be converted into glucose-6-phosphate, either directly, or after first being broken down to glucose. The hormones *insulin* and *estrogen* promote phosphorylation of blood glucose to glucose-6-phosphate. *Adrenalin* has the reverse effect, bringing about dephosphorylation of glucose.

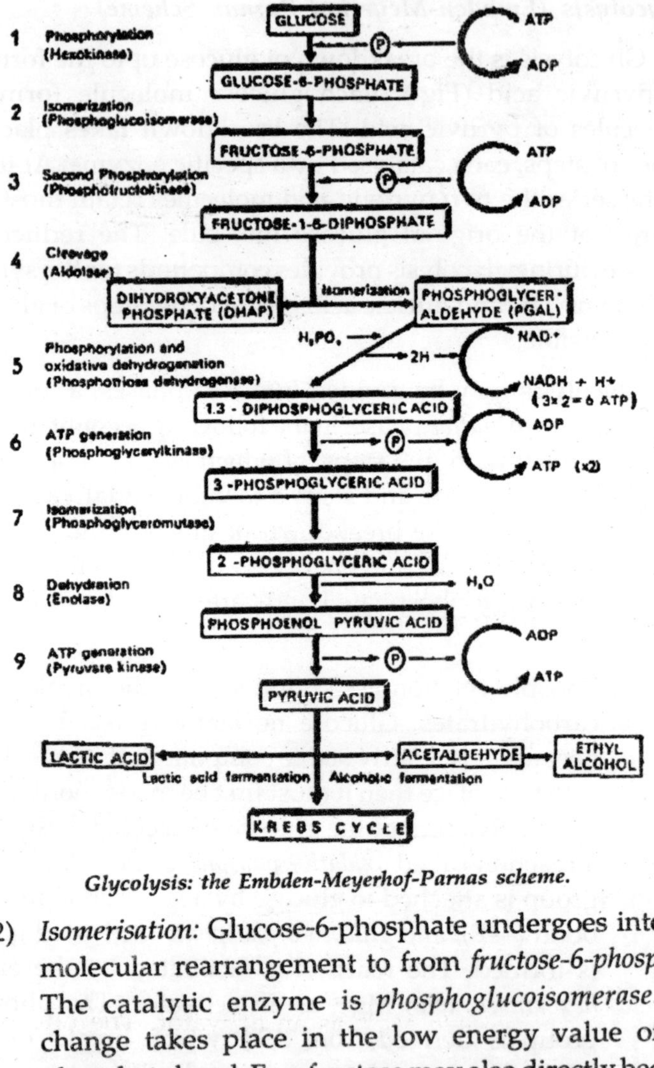

Glycolysis: the Embden-Meyerhof-Parnas scheme.

(2) *Isomerisation:* Glucose-6-phosphate undergoes internal molecular rearrangement to from *fructose-6-phosphate.* The catalytic enzyme is *phosphoglucoisomerase.* No change takes place in the low energy value of the phosphate bond. Free fructose may also directly become fructose-6-phosphate with the help of ATP.

(3) *Second Phosphorylation:* Fructose-6-phosphate undergoes phosphorylation to form *fructose-1, 6-diphosphate.* ATP is again the phosphorylating agent, while the catalytic enzyme is *phosphofructokinase.*

(4) *Cleavage:* Fructose-1, 6-diphosphate splits into two 3C halves between carbon atoms 3 and 4 under the action of the enzyme *aldolase.* The two halves *(triose phosphates)* each contain three carbon atoms, but are not identical. One half is *dihydroxyacetone phosphate* (DHAP) and the other *3-phosphoglyceraldehyde.* These molecules undergo internal rearrangement *(isomerisation)* and become identical *3-phosphoglyceraldehyde* (PGAL) molecules. The catalyzing enzyme is *triosephosphate isomerase.* In photosynthesis,PGAL is the main end product.

(5) *Phosphorylation and Oxidative Dehydrogenation:* PGAL undergoes simultaneous phosphorylation and oxidative dehydrogenation. The PGAL molecule has a phosphate group attached to one end by a low energy bond (—P). During phosphorylation, under the catalysing action of the enzyme *phosphotriose dehydrogenase,* a second phosphate group is added to the other end. The phosphorylating agent which provides the phosphate group is *phosphoric acid.* Oxidative dehydrogenation takes place simultaneously. Two hydrogen atoms are removed and are accepted by NAD^+ *(nicotinamide adenine dinucleotide),* which is converted into NADH + H^+. The newly added phosphate group acquires a high energy phosphate bond (~ P). The end product is *1, diphosphoglyceric acid,* an energy-rich compound.

(6) *ATP Generation:* 1, 3-phosphoglyceric acid now transfers its phosphate with high-energy bond to ADP, forming *3-phosphoglyceric acid* (PGA). The catalytic enzyme is *phosphoglyceryl kinase.* ADP acquires the high energy bond phosphate and becomes ATP.

(7) *Isomerisation:* The 3-phosphoglyceric acid molecule undergoes internal rearrangement and becomes *2-phosphoglyceric acid.* The catalysing enzyme is *phosphoglyceromutase.*

(8) *Dehydration:* The 2-PGA molecule loses hydrogen and oxygen in the form of water *(dehydration),* to form *phosphoenol pyruvic acid.* This step is catalysed by *enolase.* The energy is redistributed within the molecule, and the phosphate on position 2 is raised to a high-energy state. Thus a new high-energy phosphate bond is formed.

(9) *ATP Generation:* The phosphoenol pyruvic acid molecule transfers its high-energy bond phosphate to ADP, which is converted into ATP, and *pyruvic acid* is formed. Pyruvic acid does not have any phosphate groups. The reaction is catalysed by *pyruvate kinase.* It should be noted that two molecules of pyruvic acid are formed per molecule of glucose metabolised. In step 4 the *fructose-1, 6-diphosphate* molecule is cleaved into *two* triose phosphate molecules, each of which then passes through steps 5 to 9.

The Essential Features of Glycolysis are Summarised below:

(1) The starting compound is usually a 6-carbon atom glucose unit.

(2) The end product is two molecules of 3-carbon atom pyruvic acid.

(3) In the absence of oxygen pyruvic acid is converted into either *ethyl alcohol* (alcoholic fermentation)or *lactic acid* (lactic acid fermentation or muscle glycolysis).

(4) Pyruvic and lactic acids may be returned to the liver where they can be re-synthesised to form *glycose* or *glycogen* by *reverse anaerobic glycolysis.*

(5) Alternately, lactic and pyruvic acids may be broken down in the liver to yield *carbon dioxide* and *water* through the *Krebs cycle.*

(6) In all there are *four phosphorylations* during glycolysis.

Two phosphate groups are supplied by *ATP* (steps 1 and 3) and two by *phosphoric acid* (step 5).

(7) Four molecules of ATP are formed during anaerobic glycolysis (steps 6 and 9). Two molecules are, however, used up (steps 1 and 3) during the process. Therefore there is a *net gain of only two ATP molecules.*

(8) Each molecule of PGAL liberates a pair of hydrogens which are accepted by NAD^+ to form NADH + H^+ (step 5) under aerobic conditions. This pair of hydrogens is passed-down the hydrogen transport system to yield 3 molecules of ATP. Thus the two PGAL molecules formed by splitting of fructose-1, 6-diphosphate yield 6 molecules of ATP through the hydrogen transport system.

(9) The chemical bond energy from glucose is stored in ATP and NADH molecules. ATP is the main source of immediate energy for all biological processes. This energy is stored in the high-energy bond of the terminal phosphate group. When this bond is broken the terminal phosphate group separates, energy is released, and ATP is converted into ADP.

(10) Glycolysis involves oxidation without the direct use of oxygen. The oxidation is actually a process of *dehydrogenation.*

Stage II: Pyruvic Acid Oxidation

Pyruvic acid, the end product of glycolysis, does not enter the citric acid cycle directly. The 3-carbon atom molecule of pyruvic acid is first changed into a 2-carbon atom *acetic acid* molecule. One carbon is released as carbon dioxide *(decarboxylation).* Acetic acid on entering the mitochondria unites with *coenzyme A* (CoA) to form *acetyl-CoA* ('active acetate'). This reaction is catalysed by several enzymes collectively known as *pyruvate dehydrogenase.* Two hydrogen atoms are released in the reaction. They are accepted by NAD^+ to form NADH + H^+. The pair of hydrogen atoms is passed down the electron transport system and three molecules of ATP are generated. Since two pyruvic acid molecules are formed during metabolism of one molecule of glucose, in all *six* molecules of ATP are formed during oxidation of the two pyruvic acid molecules.

Stage III: Krebs Citric Acid Cycle

It has been seen that pyruvic acid is converted either into *ethyl alcohol* (alcoholic fermentation) or *lactic acid* (lactic acid fermentation or muscle glycolysis) in the absence of oxygen *(anaerobic condition)*. In the presence of oxygen *(aerobic condition)*, however, its metabolism is different. Pyruvic acid is oxidised to *acetyl-CoA*, which then undergoes a series of changes referred to as *Krebs citric acid cycle*. The citric acid cycle is also called the *tricarboxylic acid cycle* (TCA cycle) since citric acid is a tricarboxylic acid, i.e. with three-COOH groups. Each cycle results in the conversion of one molecule of acetic acid, in the form of acetyl-CoA, to carbon dioxide and water.

Formation of Citric Acid: The first step in the citric acid cycle is the condensation of the 2-carbon-atom *acetyl- CoA* with a 4-carbon atom *oxaloacetic acid* molecule to form a 6-carbon-atom molecule of *citric acid*. This reaction is irreversible. Acetyl-CoA gives its acetyl group to oxaloacetic acid to form the citric acid molecule. CoA is released and reacts with more pyruvic acid. The linkage between the acetyl group and CoA in acetyl-CoA is hydrolysed by a molecule of water. The catalysing enzyme is *citrate synthetase.*

Dehydration: Citric acid undergoes dehydration under the catalytic action of the enzyme *aconitase* to form *cis-aconitic acid* (6 carbon atoms).

Hydration: Cis-aconitic acid is rehydrated to *isocitric acid,* again under the influence of *aconitase*. The transformation of citric acid to isocitric acid is one of *isomerisation*. Citric acid can also yield isocitric acid without cis-aconitic acid occurring as a free intermediate.

Dehydrogenation I: Isocitric acid undergoes *dehydrogenation* in the presence of the enzyme *isocitrate dehydrogenase* to form *oxalo succinic acid.* The pair of hydrogen atoms removed is accepted by NAD^+ to form NADH + H^+. The occurrence of oxalosuccinic acid has been doubted by some workers. It may occur only as an enzyme-bound intermediate.

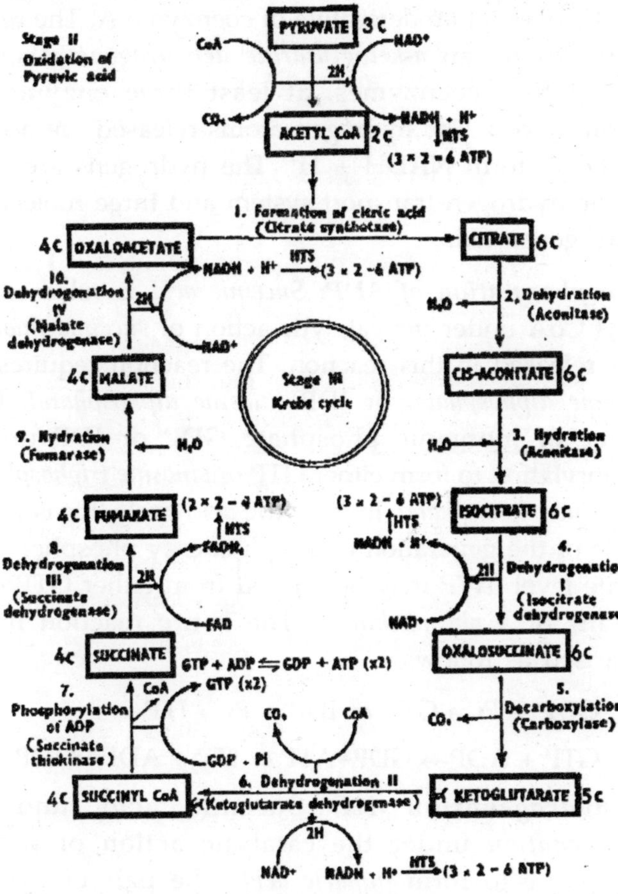

Krebs citric acid cycle. The names of the enzymes catalysing each step are given in brackets.

Decarboxylation I: Oxalosuccinic acid (or isocitric acid) undergoes *decarboxylation* to form α *-ketoglutaric acid.* One CO_2 is removed. Because of the loss of one carbon atom during *decarboxylation* the α -ketoglutaric molecule has five carbon atoms. The reaction is catalysed by *carboxylase.*

Dehydrogenation II and Carboxylation II: α -Ketoglutaric acid undergoes simultaneous *decarboxylation* and *dehydrogenation,* and joins with coenzyme A to form *succinyl-CoA,* a 4-carbon atom derivative of coenzyme A. The reaction is catalysed by an *a-ketoglutarate dehydrogenase* complex involving four coenzymes, at least three enzymes and magnesium ions. The hydrogen atoms released are accepted by NAD^+ to form NADH + H^+. The hydrogens are passed down the hydrogen transport system and three molecules of ATP are generated.

Phosphorylation of ADP: *Succinic acid* is released from succinyl CoA under the catalytic action of *succinic thiokinase.* CoA is released in this reaction. The reaction requires GDP *(guanosine diphosphate)* or IDP *(inosine diphosphate).* In the presence of inorganic phosphate GDP or IDP undergo phosphorylation to form either GTP *(guanosine triphosphate)* or ITP *(inosine triphosphate).* In the citric acid cycle this is the only example of the generation of a high-energy phosphate at the substrate level. ATP may be formed from either GTP or ITP by means of a *phosphokinase.* The entire reaction may be summarised as follows:

(i) GDP + Pi $\rightarrow$ GTP *or* IDP + Pi $\rightarrow$ ITP .

(ii) GTP + ADP $\rightarrow$ GDP+ATP *or* ITP + ADP $\rightarrow$ IDP + ATP

Dehydrogenation III: Succinic acid undergoes *dehydrogenation* under the catalytic action of *succinate dehydrogenase* to form *fumaric acid.* The pair of hydrogen atoms formed is transferred directly to *flavoprotein* without the participation of NAD^+. Flavoprotein contains FAD (flavin adenine dinucleotide) and nonhaeme iron (NHI). FAD accepts the hydrogen atoms to form $FADH_2$. Because the first ATP-generating step of the hydrogen transport system is passed over, only *two* molecules of ATP are generated per pair of hydrogen atoms when FAD is the hydrogen acceptor.

Hydration II: Fumaric acid is hydrated to form *malic* acid. The reaction is catalysed by the enzyme *fumarase.*

Dehydrogenation IV: In the final reaction malic acid is transformed into *oxalocetic acid,* which is thus regenerated. The catalytic enzyme is *malate dehydrogenase.* Dehydrogenation takes place during the process. NAD^+ accepts the hydrogen atoms to form $NADH+H^+$. The pair of hydrogens is passed down the hydrogen transport system, and three molecules of ATP are generated.

It should be noted that two molecules of pyruvic acid are formed per molecule of glucose during glycolysis. Therefore, two molecules of oxaloacetic acid per molecule of glucose are formed at the end of Krebs cycle. The fate of only one pyruvic acid molecule has been traced in the figure. The essential features of the citric acid cycle may now be summarised.

(1) The starting point for the citric acid cycle is acetyl-CoA and oxaloacetic acid.

(2) Acetyl-CoA is formed from the products of metabolism of carbohydrates (pyruvic acid), fats (fatty acids) and proteins (certain amino acids.).

(3) Oxaloacetic acid is a normal constituent of cells. It reacts with acetyl-CoA and water to form *citric acid.*

(4) Citric acid undergoes a series of degradations to form oxaloacetic acid, which re-enters the cycle.

(5) In each cycle two carbon atoms are released as carbon dioxide *(decarboxylation),* most of which is lost as a waste product.

(6) Four *dehydrogenation* reactions occur in each cycle, releasing four pairs of hydrogen atoms. Three pairs of hydrogens are accepted by NAD^+ to form $NADH + H^+$. Each pair of hydrogens when transported through the hydrogen transport system generates *three* molecules of ATP. Thus nine molecules of ATP are generated by hydrogens accepted by NAD^+. One pair of hydrogens is accepted by FAD of flavoprotein to form $FADH_2$. These hydrogens when passed through the hydrogen transport system yield only *two* molecules of ATP, since the first ATP- generating step is passed over. Thus in each Krebs cycle proper, 11 molecules of ATP are generated through the hydrogen transport system.

(7) One molecule of ATP is generated directly at the substrate level (step 7) in each cycle.

Stage IV. Oxidative Phosphorylation in the Hydrogen Transport System

Oxidation and reduction. In the 18th century Lavoisier showed that combination of inorganic materials and metabolism of living organisms were fundamentally the same processes. Both are processes of *oxidation,* in which oxygen is consumed and carbon dioxide and water produced. The definition of oxidation has since then undergone a change. In living systems *oxidation* is the *removal* of hydrogen atoms from a molecule, and *reduction* is the *addition* of hydrogen atoms. Removal of a hydrogen atom in effect means the removal of a proton and an electron.

Both oxidation and reduction go on simultaneously. When one substance releases hydrogen atoms another substance accepts them. The substance *releasing* hydrogen *(hydrogen donor)* is said to be *oxidised,* while the substance *accepting* hydrogen *(hydrogen acceptor)* is said to be *reduced.* The release of energy from a cell may be entirely independent of oxygen, as in anaerobic organisms.

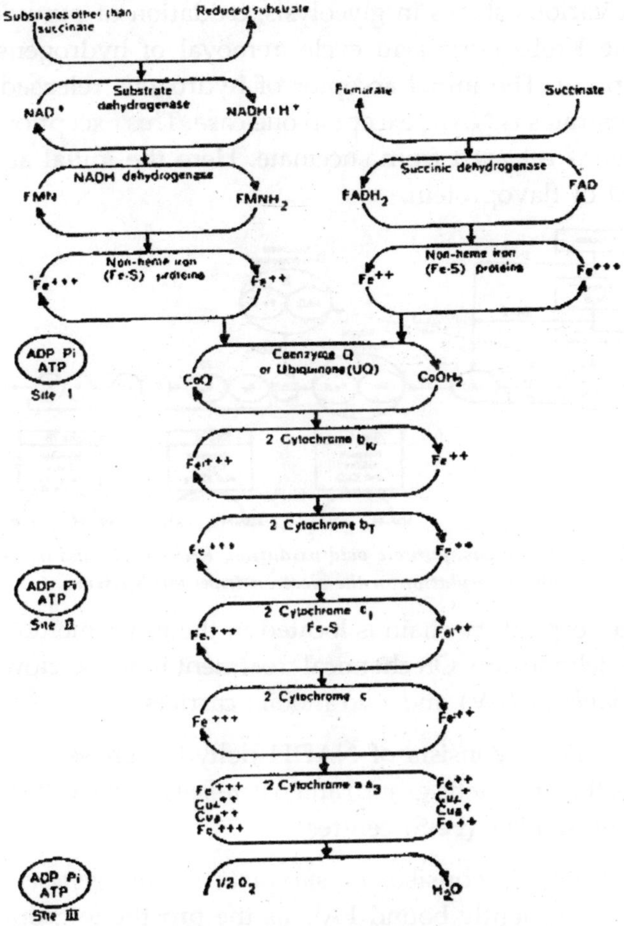

The hydrogen/electron transport system.

The electron transport system or respiratory chain. The hydrogen and electron transport system consists of several hydrogen and electron acceptors.

Biological oxidation-reduction reactions involve both hydrogen and electron acceptors. Hydrogen or electrons are passed from one acceptor to another. There are several *intermediate* hydrogen acceptors, and a *final* hydrogen acceptor which is molecular oxygen.

At various stages in glycolysis, oxidation of pyruvic acid and the Krebs citric acid cycle, removal of hydrogens (2H) takes place. The initial acceptor of hydrogens released from the substrates is NAD, except in one case. This exception is the hydrogens released from succinate. Here the initial acceptor is FAD of flavoprotein.

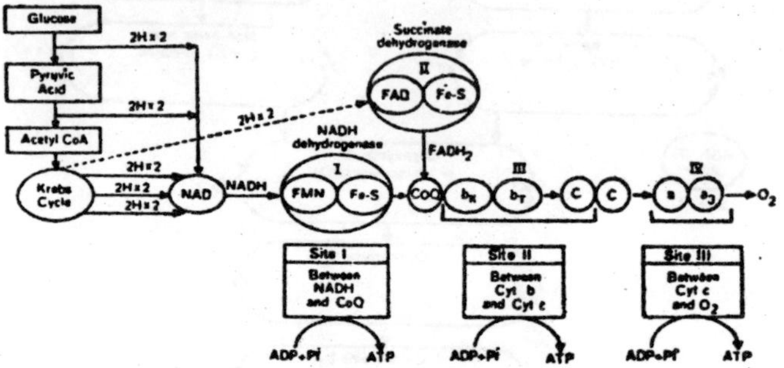

Outline of glycolysis, pyruvic acid oxidation, Krebs cycle and oxidative phosphorylation in the electron transport system.

The respiratory chain is located in the inner membrane of the mitochondrion. On chemical treatment it breaks down into five *complexes* (I-V) and two mobile carriers.

Complex I consists of NADH dehydrogenase (of which FMN is the prosthetic group) and 6 *non-heme iron (NHI) proteins* with *iron-sulphur* (Fe-S) centres.

Complex II consists of *succinate dehydrogenase* which contains covalently bound FAD as the prosthetic group, two Fe-S centres, and another Fe-S protein. Cytochrome b (absorbance 557.5 nm) has also been reported in complex II.

Between complexes II and III is the mobile carrier *coenzyme* Q(CoQ) or *ubiquinone* (UQ).

Complex III contains cytochromes b_K, b_T and c_1 and a non-heme iron protein with an Fe-S centre.

Between complexes III and IV is the mobile carrier *cytochrome c*.

Complex IV (Cytochrome c oxidase) contains cytochromes a.a_3 and two copper centres (Cuα and Cuβ)

Complex V (ATPase complex) consists of a *headpiece* (F_1, ATPase proper), a *stalk* of F_5 (OSCP) and F_6 and a *basepiece* (Fo) containing the proton channel.

Components of the Respiratory Chain

Substrate Dehydrogenases (Nicotinamide Nucleotide Dehydrogenases): Biological oxidations are catalysed by *enzymes* which function in conjunction with *coenzymes* or electron carries. The *nicotinamide nucleotides* are *coenzymes* for dehydrogenases (enzymes). They are also referred to as the *pyridine nucleotides* because nicotinamide is a *substituted pyridine.*

The substrate dehydrogenases contain either *nicotinamide adenine dinucleotide* (NAD) or *nicotinamide adenine dinucleotide phosphate* (NADP), a phosphorylated form of NAD (Figs.). The old name for NAD was *diphosphopyridine nucleotide* (DPN) or *coenzyme I,* and that for NADP was *triphosphopyridine nucleotide* (TPN) or *coenzyme II.* NAD and NADP act as hydrogen carriers through alternate reduction and oxidation of the pyridine ring. The reduced coenzymes are NADH and NADPH, respectively. In general, NAD serves as an *oxidizing agent* by accepting hydrogen from substrates. NADP on the other hand is more often used as a *reducing agent* in biosynthetic processes, and

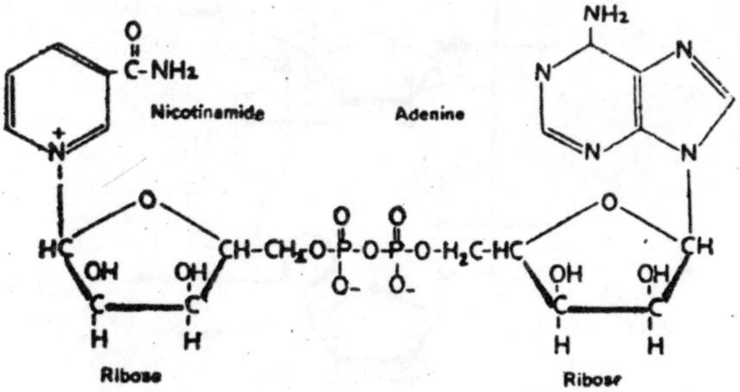

Nicotinamide adenine dinucleotide (NAD^+) or diphosphopyridine nucleotide (DPN^+).

is reduced to NADPH. NAD and NADP act as coenzymes. They are essential for enzyme activity, but easily dissociate from the apoprotein. On doing so they lose their biological activity.

NAD consists of two nucleotides, *nicotinamide ribose phosphate* and *adenine ribose phosphate:* hence the name nicotinamide adenine disphosphate. The reactive part of the NAD molecule is the *nicotinamide ring.*

The N of nicotinamide is positively charged, and so NAD is also written as NAD^+. NAD is the major electron acceptor of dehydrogenation reactions in which a pair of hydrogens (2H) are released. The two hydrogens consist of two protons (H^+) and two electrons (e^-). Since NAD^+ already has a positive charge, it accepts only one hydrogen proton (H^+) and two electrons, the equivalent of a *hydride ion.* The second proton is lost to the surrounding medium in which it is soluble. NAD^+ is reduced to NADH + H^+.

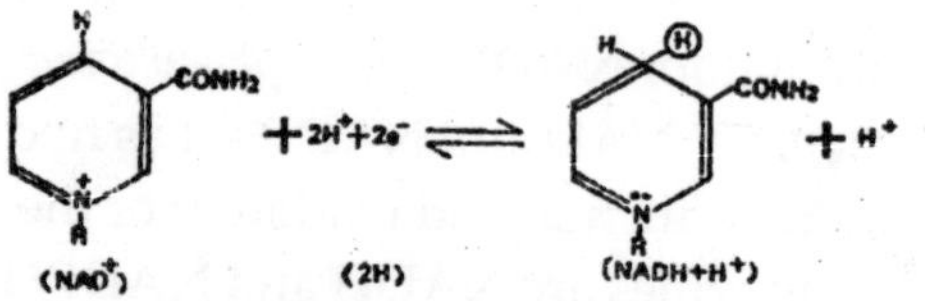

B. NAD+ on accepting 2H becomes NADH + H+. One hydrogen is accepted by NAD+ and the other is released as a hydrogen ion (H+).

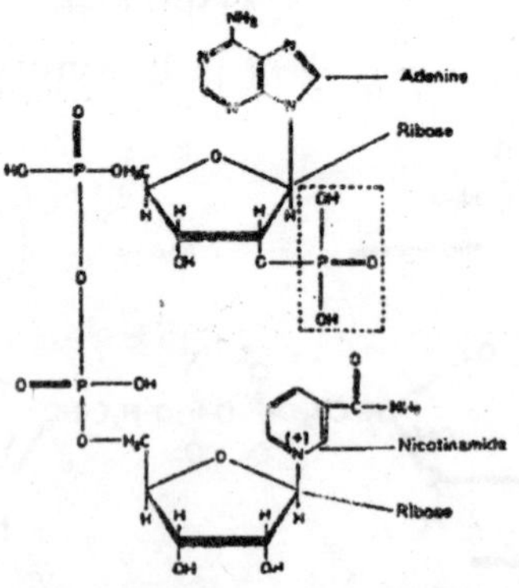

Nicotinamide adenine dinucleotide phosphate ($NADP^+$). When a phosphate group is added to NAD it becomes $NADP^+$.

$$NAD^+ + 2H \rightarrow NADH + H^+$$

$$\text{or } NAD^+ + (2H^+ + 2e^-) \rightarrow NADH + H^+$$

While writing, the H^+ is often omitted and the reduced form is written as NADH. Sometimes it is also written as $NADH_2$.

NADP has a phosphate group instead of the 2'- hydroxyl group of NAD. On accepting 2H it is reduced to NADPH + H^+.

$$NADP + 2H \rightarrow NADPH + H^+$$

NADPH is the electron donor in most reductive biosyntheses, while NADH is mainly used for ATP generation.

Flavoproteins: Both complexes I and II contain dehydrogenases. Complex I contains *NADH dehydrogenase* while complex II contains *succinic deyhdrogenase.* These dehydrogenases contain *flavoproteins* as the main redox component, and also one or more *iron sulphur (Fe-S) proteins.*

The flavoprotein of complex I (FP_N) consists of an *apoprotein* plus tightly bound *flavin mononucleotide* (FMN) as its *prosthetic group.* The flavoprotein of succinic dehydrogenase (FPs) contains *flavin adenine dinucleotide* (FAD) as the prosthetic group. Since both FMN and FAD are tightly bound to their apoproteins, they act as prosthetic groups rather than as coenzymes.

FAD consists of two halves, *flavin mononucleotide* (FMN) and *adenosine monophosphate* (AMP) (Fig.). The components of FAD are *flavin D-ribitol, D-ribose, adenine* and two *phosphates.* A break between the two phosphates results in FMN and *adenine D-ribose phosphate* (AMP). *Flavin D-ribitol* contains a three-ringed *isoalloxazine* nucleus, which is the reactive part. In contrast to NAD^+, this nucleus can accept both hydrogens ($2H = 2H^+ + 2e^-$) released by the substrate molecule. FAD on accepting the hydrogens is reduced to $FADH_2$.

$$FAD + 2H \rightarrow FADH_2$$

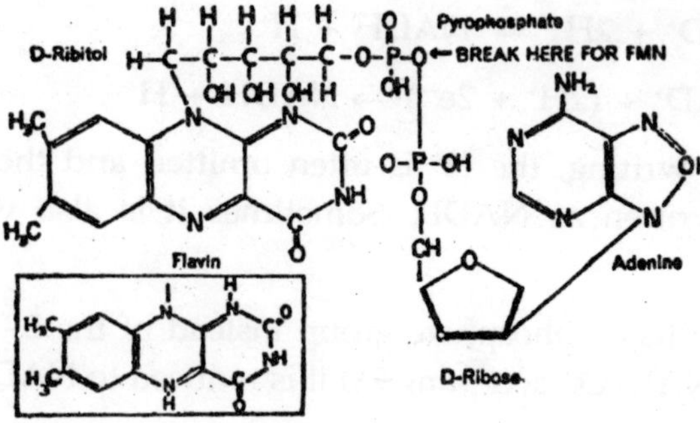

Flavin adenine dinucleotide (FAD). FAD consists of two halves, flavin mononucleotide (FMN), shown on the left, and adenosine monophosphate (AMP), shown on the right. Inset: FMN on accepting (2H) is reduced to $FMNH_2$.

However, it is possible that *in vivo* the nucleus carries only one reducing equivalent. It would thus oscillate in the *semiquinone form* between the oxidised and the reduced forms. FMN on accepting 2H from $NADH + H^+$ is reduced to $FMNH_2$.

$$NADH + H^+ + FMN \rightarrow FMNH_2 + NAD^+$$

The standard redox potential of the $FADH_2$ /FAD couple is -210 mV and that of the $FMNH_2$ /FMN couple -190 mV. These values are, however, different when the flavins are bound to the apoprotein. NADH dehydrogenase. This enzyme is also called *NADH: CoQ reductase* and is located in complex I. It consists of *flavoprotein*, which has *flavin mononucleotide* (FMN) as its prosthetic group, *iron-sulphur* (Fe-S) centres. The molecular weight of the enzyme is about 550,000.

Succinic dehydrogenase (MW 70,000) is found in complex II. It contains covalently bound FAD as the prosthetic group and two Fe-S centres (Fe-S S1 and Fe-S S2). The FAD is covalently bound to the apoprotein through a *histidine* (His) residue. This covalent linkage permits raising of the standard redox potential of $FADH_2$/FAD from that of the free form (—210 mV) to that of succinate / fumarate (+30 mV). An additional Fe-S protein (MW 27,000) designated as Fe-S S3 is associated with succinic dehydrogenase to from complex II (succinate-CoQ reductase).

Iron-sulphur Proteins (Fe-S): Some enzymes use metallic ions linked to the apoenzyme for transfer of electrons in oxidation-reduction reactions. Such enzymes are called *Metalloproteins.* The commonly involved ions are those of *iron* and *copper*. Proteins that bind iron atoms in a lattice of sulphur atoms are called *non-heme iron proteins* (NHI) or *Iron-sulphur proteins* (Fe-S). (Proteins containing iron related to a *porphyrin* group are called *heme proteins).* Complex I contains 6 iron-sulphur centres, Fe-S Nla, Fe-S Nlb, Fe-S N2, Fe-S N3, Fe-S N4 and Fe-S N5, the 'N' indicating that the centre is a part of NADH dehydrogenase. There is a large difference in the E°' values of centres N1, N3, N4, N5 ($\leq$—260 mV) and N2 (-20 mV). This indicates that electron transfer from (N1, N3, N4, N5) $\rightarrow$ N2 releases sufficient energy to synthesise ATP.

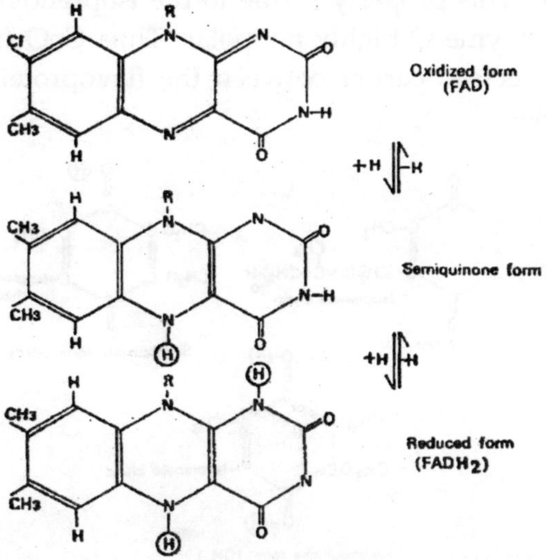

Structure of the reactive, 3-ringed isoalloxazine nucleus of flavin adenine dinucleotide (FAD) during oxidised, semiquinone and reduced states.

The non-heme iron in *succinate dehydrogenase* (complex II) is found in three centres, Fe-S S1, Fe-S S2 and Fe-S S3. The 'S' indicates that the centres are found in succinate dehydrogenase. Electron transfer probably takes place in the following direction :

FAD→ Fe-S S1→ Fe-S S3. The E°′ of Fe-S S2 is too low for it to be catalytically active. Complex III also contains a non-heme iron protein (NHI) (MW 26,000) which has the iron-sulphur (Fe-S) centre.

Coenzyme Q (CoQ) or Ubiquinone (UQ)

Coenzyme Q is an electron carrier which is strictly speaking not an enzyme. It is a lipid-soluble quinone acting as a coenzyme. Structurally it has a *benzoquinone* nucleus attached to an unsaturated *isoprenoid* side chain (Fig.). The number of isoprenoid units varies from 6 to 10 (CoQ_{6-10}). Bacteria typically contains 6 isoprenoid units, and this number is also found in some yeasts. Mammalian mitochondria contains 10 units. Coenzyme Q is able to diffuse rapidly in the mitochondrial membrane. This property is due to the isoprenoid tail which makes coenzyme Q highly nonpolar. Thus CoQ functions as a mobile electron carrier between the flavoproteins and the cytochromes.

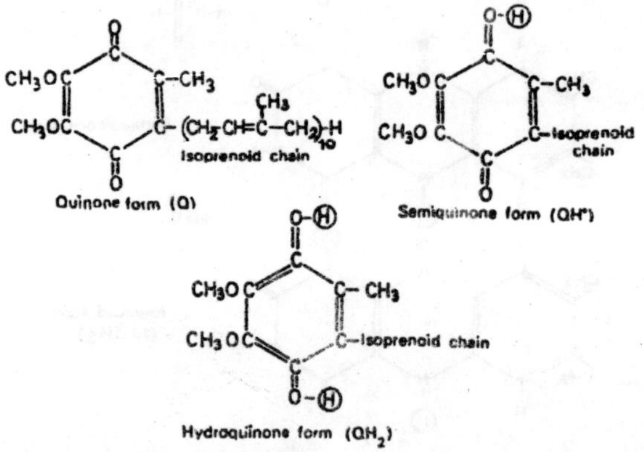

Coenzyme Q (CoQ) or ubiquinone (UQ).

A. *Quinone form (Q). Fully oxidised. Both oxygens connected to the ring by double bonds.*

B. *Semiquinone form (QH·). Semi-oxidised. Hydrogen atom attached to one oxygen.*

C. *Hydroquinone form (QH_2). Fully reduced. Hydrogen atoms attached to both oxygens.*

Coenzyme Q is found in the mitochondria in the oxidised *quinone* form under aerobic conditions and in the reduced *quinol* form under anaerobic conditions. The reduced form is called *hydroquinone* ($CoQH_2$) or *dihydroxyubiquinone.* The partially reduced form is called *semiquinone.* It is relatively stable and can transfer one electron. Thus CoQ can take part in both one-electron transfer reactions *(semiquinone)* and two-electron transfers *(hydroquinone).*

Plastoquinone, which occurs in chloroplast and functions in photosynthesis, is closely related to coenzyme Q. It contains two CH_3 groups which replace the methoxyl ($-OCH_3$) groups of coenzyme Q. In some bacterial respiratory systems *menaquinone* takes the place of coenzyme Q. The polyisoprenoid side chain is also present in vitamins E and K.

The Cytochromes

In 1925, Keilin gave the name 'cytochromes' to certain conjugated proteins. He identified three cytochromes which he named a, b and c. Since then about 50 cytochromes have been identified. They are named according to which of the original three they resemble e.g. a_1, a_3, c_1, c_2, c_3, etc. Three main types of cytochromes, the b-, c- and a-types, have been distinguished in the mammalian respiratory chain. There are at least two b-type cytochromes, *cyt* b_K (after Keilin) and *cyt* b_T (transduing). The main c-type cytochromes are *cyt c* and *cyt* c_1. The a-type cytochromes include *cyt* $a.a_3$. *(cytochrome oxidase)*

*The cytochromes are conjugat*ed proteins consisting of an *apoprotein* and a *prosthetic group (heme).* The heme consists of a *porphyrin* with a central *iron* atom. The porphyrins are complex carbon-nitrogen molecules that usually surround a metal ion (Me) to from *metalloporphyrins* (Fig.). The metal ion is magnesium in chlorophyll and iron in cytochromes and haemoglobin. Porphyrins are cyclic compounds consisting of 4 *pyrrole rings* linked by methylene bridges. The H substituted positions of the ring are named 1 to 8. The methylene bridges are called α, β, γ and δ.

Heme (iron protoporphyrin IX) is the prosthetic group of cytochromes b, c_1, c, myoglobin and haemoglobin (Table). In cytochromes c and c_1 the heme is covalently attached to the protein by *thioether linkages.*

$$\begin{array}{c} \quad CH_3 \\ \quad | \\ R\text{—}CH\text{—}S\text{—}CH_2\text{—}R' \end{array}$$

In cytochrome b, the heme is not covalently bonded to protein. The iron-porphyrin prosthetic group of cytochromes a and a_3 is called *heme A*. Heme A has a formyl group instead of one of the methyl groups of heme in cytochromes c and c_1, and the vinyl group is replaced by a hydrocarbon group (long hydrophobic isoprenoid chain).

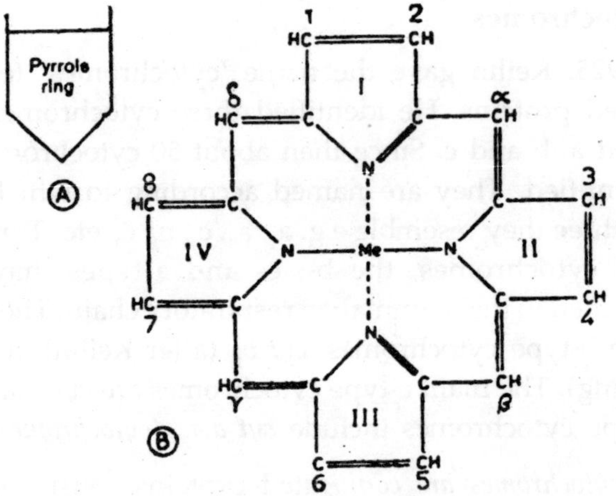

General structure of a porphyrin.

The substituent groups on carbons 2, 4, 5 and 8 of heme differ in the different cytochromes.

Ionic iron exists in two forms, Fe^{++} (ferrous) and Fe^{+++} (ferric). One form can be converted into the other by loss or gain of an electron.

$$\underset{\text{(Ferric)}}{Fe^{+++}} \underset{\text{-e, Oxidation}}{\overset{\text{Reduction, +e}}{\rightleftarrows}} \underset{\text{(Ferrous)}}{Fe^{++}}$$

Structure of Heme

Heme	Carbon-2	Carbon-4	Carbon-5	Carbon-8
a	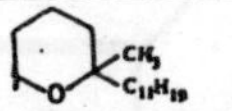	$-CH=CH_2$	-	-CHO
b (protoheme)	$-CH=CH_2$	$-CH=CH_2$	$-CH_3$	CH_3
c (mesoheme)	$-CH \cdot CH_3$ with S-protein	$-CH \cdot CH_3$ with S-protein	$-CH_3$	$-CH_3$

The Fe in the cytochrome molecule acts as an electron donor or acceptor. After *accepting* electrons the atom is *reduced,* while after *donating* electrons it is *oxidised.*

Cytochromes b: Complex III contains at least two b-type cytochromes, cytochrome b_K (cyt_{560}) and *cytochrome* b_T (cyt b_{565}). The subscripts K and T stand for *Keilin-type* cytochrome b and *transducing* cytochromes b, respectively. The two cytochromes are either located in the middle of the membrane, or according to another view, they span the membrane. The $E^{\circ\prime}$ of cyt b_T is ATP-variable. It changes from —30 mV in the absence of ATP to + 245 mV in the presence of a high ATP concentration. It is therefore possible that cyt b_T plays a direct role in energy conservation. The $E^{o\prime}$ of cytocrome b_K does not vary with ATP, and cyt b_K probably acts as a simple redox carrier. The b cytochrome contain *protoheme,* which is also found in bacterial cytochrome c.

Cytochrome c (Fig.): The cytochromes c include the eukaryote mitochondrial *cyt c,* the bacterial photosynthetic *cyt* c_2 and several others of prokaryotic origin. They are not enzymes in the conventional sense but are cofactors for the proteins with which they interact. The single heme prosthetic group is bound to the polypeptide chain of 82 to 134 residues near the amino terminus.

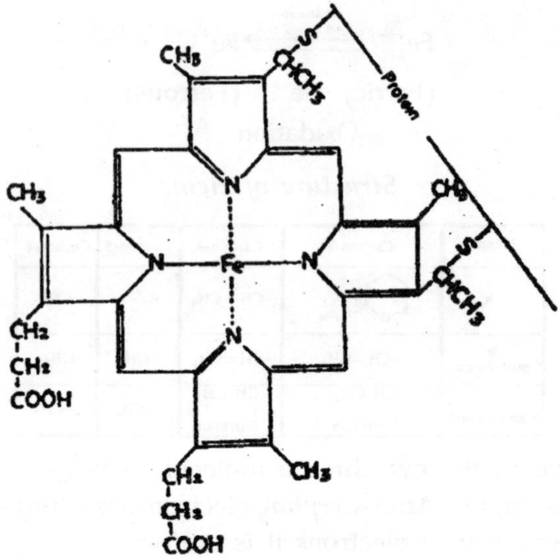

Cytocrome c.

The molecular weight of cytochrome c is about 12,600 (104 amino acids). The standard redox potential (E°′) is +254 mV for isolated cyt c and +235 mV in mitochondria. The heme group *(heme c, mesoheme)* is covalently bound to the polypeptide chain via thioether linkages from C—2 and C—4. There is also coordinate linkage between heme and His-18 and Met-80 of the polypetide chain.

The polypeptide chain is wound around the heme backbone. The heme is inserted into a hydrophobic slit within the protein in such a way that only parts of pyrrole rings I and IV are exposed. The amino acid sequences of the polypeptide chain of over 50 species has been determined. There are 28 invariant positions in the peptide chain.

Cytochrome c_1 is an intrinsic protein with MW 30,6000 (from beef heart mitochondria). Unlike *cyt c, it* appears to be firmly bound to the membrane. The heme-containing part of *cytochrome* c_1 is located on the C-side of the membrane from where it can easily transfer electrons to *cyt c.*

Cytochromes. a_3 (Cytochrome c Oxidase): Although cytochromes a and a_3 are considered to be separate cytochromes they have never been physically separated, and apparently cannot function independently. The functional unit of mammalian cytochrome oxidase consists of two *heme molecules* and two *copper atoms* (Cuα and Cuβ). Cytochrome a does not react with carbon monoxide and is therefore not inhibited by it. Cytochrome a_3 on the other hand reacts with CO and is inhibited by it. CO competes with oxygen for the binding site on the ferrous ion. The cytochrome oxidase complex is oriented perpendicularly to the plane of the membrane. It is about 83A long, and therefore extends considerably beyond the 40-50A lipid bilayer. The complex spans the membrane with cytochrome a on the C-side and cytochrome a_3 on the membrane side.

Beef heart cytochrome oxidase consists of 6 subunits, I (MW 40,000, II (MW 22,500), III (MW 15,000), IV (MW 11,200), V (MW 9,800) and VI (MW 7,000). Subunits II, V and VI face the C-side of the membrane, I and IV are in the middle and III on the M-side. Cyctochrome c oxidase contains four units (cyt a, Cyt a_3, Cuα and Cuβ) which carry one electron each. Thus four electrons are stored in the enzyme prior to discharge. The four electrons (4e⁻) combine with four protons ($4H^+$) and one molecule of oxygen to form water.

$$4H^+ + 4e^- + O_2 \rightarrow 2H_2O$$

Standard Oxidation-reduction Potentials of the Components of the Respiratory Chain

Components	*From C.W. Jones (1976)*	*From Wilson et al (1972,76)*
Lactate/Pyruvate		—0.185 V
Succinate/Fumarate	+ 30 mV	+0.031 V
NADH/NAD^+	—320 mV	—0.320 V
NADPH/NADP	—324 mV	

Contd...

Components	*From C.W. Jones (1976)*	*From Wilson et al (1972,76)*
$FMNH_2/FMN$	—190 mV	
$FADH_2/FAD$	—210 mV (free)	
	+ 30 mV (+apoprotein)	~ — 0.045 V
Fe-S N1, Ee-S N3, Fe-S N4	≥—245 mV	
Fe-S N2	— 20 mV	
Fe-S S1	+ 15 mV	
Fe-S S2	—260 mV	
Fe-S S3	+ 60 mV	
CoQ or UQ	≃ — 0 mV	+0. 10 V (isolated) +0.045 V
Cyt b_T (b565)	—30 mV	—0.030 V
Cyt b_T + ATP	+240 mV	+0.245 V
Cyt b_K (b562)	+ 65 mV	+0.030 V
Fe-S	....	+ 0. 28 V
Cyt c_1	+220 mV	+ 0.215 V
Cyt c	+254 mV	+0.254 V (isolated)
Cyt a	+ 230 mV	+0. 29 V (isolated) +0.210 V
Cyt a_3	+ 375 mV	+ 0.385 V + 0.155 V(+ATP)
Cu α and Cu β	+280 mV	+0.245 V
$H_2O/½ O_2$	+ 820 mV	+ 0.815 V

The figures represent mid-point potentials ($E^{0'}$). The $E^{0'}$ value of cyt b_T changes from —0.030 V in the absence of ATP to +0.245 V in presence of high ATP concentrations. However, $E^{0'}$ for cyt a_3 drops from+0.385 V to 0.155 V in the presence of ATP.

The rodex potential (Table). The tendency for release and acceptance of electrons is called the *redox potential* ($E^{0\prime}$). The term 'redox' has been derived from reduction-oxidation. The redox potential is the *ratio of the reduced form to the oxidised form*, and is expressed in volts or millivolts. The redox potentials of various compounds of the hydrogen transport system at pH 7 are given in Table.

Transfer of hydrogen and electrons. As mentioned previously, hydrogen atoms are transferred from the substance to be oxidised to NAD^+. From NAD^+ the hydrogen atoms are transferred to FMN and CoQ. The hydrogen atom undergoes ionisation, i.e. it is split into an *electron* and a *proton*. In further stages there is no longer a transfer of hydrogens but of electrons. The electrons pass from coenzyme Q to cytochromes b_K, b_T, c_1, c, a and a_3. The protons are released free. The sequence of compounds in the hydrogen transport system is as follows.

NAD → FMN → Fe-S → CoQ → C_Yt b_K → C_Yt b_T → C_Yt c_1 → C_Yt c → C_Yt a .a_3

As the hydrogen atoms or electrons pass down the chain there is simultaneous oxidation of one coenzyme and a reduction of another at each step. The compounds of the electron transfer system first act as *oxidizing* agents by *accepting* electrons/hydrogens and then as *reducing agents* by *donating* them. Each substance in the respiratory chain is alternately oxidised and reduced. In the case of $NADH_2$ and $FMNH_2$ oxidation takes place by loss *of hydrogen*. For coenzyme Q and the cytochromes b_K, b_T, c_1, c, a and a_3, oxidation takes place by loss of electrons. At a time *two* electrons are released. Cytochromes b_K, b_T c_1, c, a and a_3 *can accept only one electron at a time*. Therefore, the electrons are captured by *two* molecules each of the enzymes of the cytochrome system.

After transfer from cytochrome a_3 an electron and a proton are brought together. They combine to produce hydrogen. The final hydrogen acceptor is molecular oxygen and H_2O is the final product. *It is because oxygen is used as the final acceptor in the hydrogen transport system that most organisms require oxygen in order to survive.*

Sites of Oxidative Phosphorylation (ATP Generation): In 1941 S. Ochoa obtained the first reliable measurement of the P/O ratio. This ratio is the number of moles of ATP generated per atom of oxygen utilised in respiration, and is used as an index of oxidative phosphorylation. The P/O ratio is also equal to the number of moles of ATP formed per pair of electrons passing down the electron transport system.

Lehninger (1951) showed that oxidation of NAD^+-linked substrates (e.g. β -hydroxybutyrate) gave a P/O ratio of about 3. This indicated that there were 3 energy coupling sites between NADH and molecular oxygen. The aerobic oxidation of one mole of NADH through the mitochondrial respiratory chain gives rise to the synthesis of 3 moles of ATP from ADP and Pi. Complex I, III and IV each contain one energy coupling site which can interact with the ATP synthesizing system.

The P/O ratio of flavin linked substrates, e.g. *succinate,* was about 2. Thus there are only two energy-coupling sites involved when succinate is the acceptor. The first energy coupling site (i. e. complex I) is bypassed. This suggested that site I of oxidative phosphorylation was located between NADH and coenzyme Q.

Lehninger (1949) used tetramethyl phenylene diamine (TMPD) to introduce electrons at cytochrome c. Studies in which cytochrome c was directly used as an electron donor showed that only one ATP was generated, since sites I and II were bypassed. This indicated that site III was to the right of cytochrome c.

Slater (1955) showed that passage of electrons from succinate to cytochrome c gave a P/O ratio of only 1. This indicated that one ATP was generated at site II.

By such experiments it has been possible to localise the three energy coupling sites as follows:

Site I—between NADH and CoQ.

Site II—between cytochormes b and c.

Site III—between cytochrome c and O_2.

A general agreement about the stoichiometric relationships of the respiratory chain components is that for every two molecules of cytochrome c there is one of complex III, two of complex IV and 16 molecules of coenzyme Q (Slater, 1967). Inhibitor binding studies (Slater, 1972) indicate that there is only one ATP synthetase (complex V) for every complex III. Thus for every *three coupling sites* of each electron transfer chain there is only one ATP synthesizing and hydrolyzing unit.

Synthesis of ATP in the presence of oxygen is called *oxidative phosphorylation*. The normal site of oxidative phosphorylation in plant and animal cells is the mitochondrion. The term oxidative phosphorylation is used because ATP production requires oxygen in the last step of the series.

It is now possible to calculate the total number of ATP molecules produced when a molecule of glucose is metabolised through glycolysis and the Krebs cycle to produce carbon dioxide and water. (Tables) Outline of ATP production during aerobic oxidation of glucose to CO_2 and H_2O.

Glycolysis

(i) ATP produced directly .... 4 molecules.

ATP used .... 2 molecules.

Net gain .... 2 molecules.

(ii) From hydrogens produced and sent down the hydrogen transport system (2 × 3) .... 6 molecules.

Pyruvic Acid Oxidation

(i) From hydrogens produced and sent down the hydrogen transport system (2 × 3) .... 6 molecules.

Krebs Cycle

(i) ATP produced directly .... 2 molecules.

(ii) From hydrogens accepted by NAD (3×3) — 9 molecules

Therefore for the two molecules of citric acid metabolised (9 × 2) .... 18 molecules.

(iii) From hydrogens accepted by FAD (1 × 2)—2 molecules.

Therefore for the two molecules of citric acid metabolised (2 × 2) .... 4 molecules.

TOTAL 38 molecules.

ATP produced during complete oxidation of one molecule of glucose to carbon dioxide and water under aerobic conditions. Glycolysis

---

(i) ATP produced by oxidation at substrate level.

Step 6. 1, 3, diphosphoglyceric acid to 3, phosphoglyceric acid (1 x 2=2)	2 ATP
Step 9. Phosphoenol pyruvic acid to pyruvic acid (1 x 2 = 2)	2 ATP
	4 ATP

ATP consumed.

Step 1. Glucose to glucose-6-phosphate	1 ATP
Step 3. Fructose-6-phosphate to fructose 1-6 diphosphate	1 ATP
NET GAIN OF ATP (4 minus 2)	2 ATP

(ii) ATP from hydrogens produced and sent down the hydrogen transport system.

Step 5. PGAL to 1, 3 diphosphoglyceric acid (3 x 2=6) 6 ATP

Total Atp Produced During Aerobic Glycolysis 8 ATP

Pyruvic Acid Oxidation

ATP from hydrogens produced and sent down the hydrogen transport system.

Pyruvic acid to acetyl CoA (3 x 2 = 6) 6 ATP

Krebs Citric Acid Cycle

ATP produced by oxidation at substrate level.

Step 7. Succinyl CoA to succinic acid (1 x 2=2)2 ATP

ATP from hydrogens produced and sent down the hydrogen transport system.

Step 4. Isocitric acid to oxalosuccinic acid, NAD acceptor, (3 x 2=6) 6 ATP

Step 6. α -ketoglutaric acid to succinyl CoA, NAD acceptor, (3 x 2 = 6) 6 ATP

Step 8. Succinic acid to fumaric acid, FAD acceptor, (2 x 2 = 4) 4 ATP

Step 10. Malic acid to oxaloacetic acid. NAD acceptor, (3 x 2 = 6) 6 ATP

24 ATP

Total ATP Produced 38 ATP

Substances Consumed and Produced during Different Stages of Respiration

	Stage I *Glycolysis*	*Stage II* *Pyruvic Acid Oxidation*	*Stage III* *Krebs Cycle*	*Stage IV* *Oxidative Phosphory-lation*	*Total*
		Substances consumed			
Glucose or products	Glucose	2 Pyruvic acids	2 Acetyl CoA	—	$C_6H_{12}O_6$
O_2	—	—	—	$6O_2$	$6O_2$
ADP	2 ADP	—	2 ADP	34 ADP	38 ADP
P	2P	—	2 P	34 P	38 P
H	—	—	—	24 H	—
CoA	—	2 CoA	—	—	—
H_2O	—	—	6 H_2O	—	—
		Substances produced			
Glucose or products	2 Pyruvic acid	2 Acetyl CoA	—	—	—
ATP	2 ATP	—	2 ATP	34 ATP	38 ATP
H	4H	4 H	16 H	—	—
CO_2	—	2 CO_2	4 CO_2	—	6 CO_2
CoA	—	—	2 CoA	—	—
H_2	—	—	—	12 H_2O	6 H_2O

Equations of the different stages of cell respiration.

(1) Stage I, Glycolysis ;

Glucose + 2 ADP + 2P $\rightarrow$ 2 Pyruvic acid + 2 ATP + 4H

(2) Stage II, Pyruvic Acid Oxidation:

2 Pyruvic acid + 2 CoA $\rightarrow$ 2 Acetyl CoA + $2CO_2$ + 4H

(3) Stage III, Krebs Citric Acid Cycle:

2 Acetyl CoA + $6H_2O$ + 2ADP+2P $\rightarrow$ $4CO_2$ + 2ATP+16H + 2CoA

(4) Stage IV, Oxidative Phosphorylation:

$$24H + 6O_2 + 34ADP + 34P \rightarrow 12H_2O + 34\ ATP$$

(5) Net Equation of Glucose Oxidation:

$$C_6H_{12}O_6 + 6O_2 + 38\ ADP + 38P \rightarrow 6CO_2 + 6H_2O + 38\ ATP$$

Energy Relationships During Cell Respiration

(Fig.). One mole (180 gm) of glucose yields about 686,000 calories on complete combustion to carbon dioxide and water. The terminal phosphate group (~) of a mole of ATP contains about 10,000 calories. Therefore the 38 molecules of ATP represent an energy yield of 380,000 calories. This is 55% of the 686,000 calories originally present in glucose. Under aerobic conditions glycolysis (glucose to pyruvic acid) releases 50,000 calories, or 7% of the total 686,000 calories free energy change. The remaining 93% is released during oxidation of pyruvic acid to acetyl CoA, the Krebs cycle and oxidation by the hydrogen transport system.

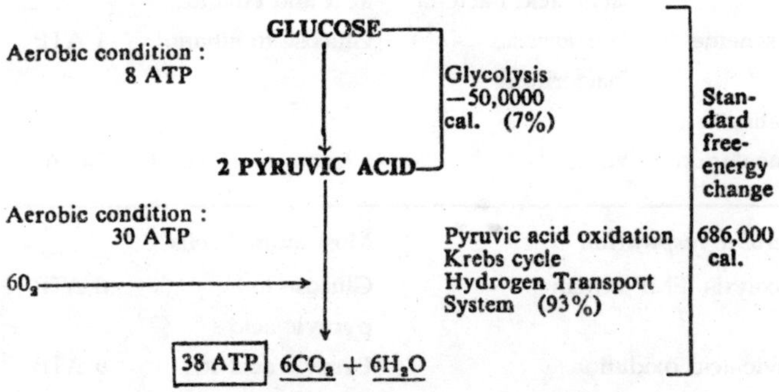

Energy relationships during cell respiration.

Organisms which do not have hydrogen transport systems do not require oxygen and are said to be *anaerobic*. Their mode of respiration is called *fermentation* and results in various products like ethanol, lactic acid and glycerol. During fermentation, glycolysis may take place by the EMP pathway, HMP pathway ED pathway, or other pathways. Organisms which have the hydrogen transport system require oxygen as the final hydrogen acceptor are said to be *aerobic.* In these organisms *aerobic glycolysis* takes place by the EMP pathway, and pyruvic acid enters the Krebs citric acid cycle.

The number of molecules of ATP produced differs in different types of respiration (Table). In anaerobic respiration the number of molecules of ATP formed is much less than in aerobic respiration.

ATP Production in different Types of Respiration

Type of Respiration	*Organism or Tissue*	*Substrate and Products*	*ATP Generated*
Fermentation (Anaerobic)			
1. EMP scheme	Yeast	Glucose to ethanol	2 ATP
2. EMP scheme	Homofermentative lactic acid bacteria	Glucose to lactic acid	2 ATP
3. HMP scheme	Heterofermentative lactic acid bacteria	Glucose to lactic acid and ethanol	1 ATP
4. ED scheme	*Pseudomonas* (bacterium)	Glucose to ethanol	1 ATP
5. Alkaline fermentation	Yeast	Glucose to glycerol	No ATP
Aerobic respiration		Most animal cells	
1. Glycolysis, EMP scheme		Glucose to pyruvic acid	8 ATP
2. Pyruvic acid oxidation		Pyruvic acid to acetyl CoA (X2)	6 ATP
3. Krebs cycle		Citric acid to oxaloacetic acid, CO_2 and H_2O (X2)	24 ATP
			38 ATP
Muscle glycolysis			
1. EMP scheme (anaerobic)	Muscle	Glycogen to lactic acid	3 ATP

Muscle respiration Muscle ***(aerobic)***		
1. Glycolysis (aerobic) EMP scheme	Glycogen to pyruvic acid	9 ATP
2. Pyruvic acid oxidation	Pyruvic acid to acetyl CoA (X2)	6 ATP
3. Krebs cycle	Citric acid to oxaloacetic acid.	24 ATP
	CO_2 and H_2O (X2)	39 ATP

During anaerobic glycolysis through the EMP pathway (e.g. yeast, and homofermentative lactic acid bacteria) there is a net gain of only 2 molecules of ATP per molecule of glucose metabolised. (2) During glycolysis through the HMP pathway (e.g. heterofermentative lactic acid bacteria) and the ED pathway (e.g. *Pseudomonas)* there is a net gain of only one molecule of ATP. (3) During alkaline fermentation in yeast no ATP is produced (Table).

When a molecule of glucose is completely metabolised to carbon dioxide and water under aerobic conditions, 38 molecules of ATP are produced: 8 during glycolysis, 6 during oxidation of pyruvic acid to acetyl CoA and 24 during the Krebs cycle.

In muscle glycolysis the initial substrate is not free glucose but *glycogen* (Fig.). Glycogen is phosphorylated by phosphoric acid and not by ATP. Thus instead of 2 ATP molecules only one is consumed. The net gain of ATP at the end of anaerobic glycolysis is therefore 4–1 = 3 ATP molecules. Under aerobic conditions 3+6=9 molecules of ATP are produced. The total ATP yield when glycogen is the initial source of glycolysis is therefore 39 molecules.

In muscle glycolysis, lactic acid is produced under anaerobic conditions. Under aerobic conditions, glucose derived from glycogen is metabolised to carbon dioxide and water. However, recent work has shown that *even under fully aerobic conditions some lactic acid is produced.* Under anaerobic conditions, lactic acid production is much larger, as much as 150 to 200 times more than the basal rate.

GLYCOGEN
Phosphorylase ↓ **nH_3PO_4**
n GLUCOSE-1-PHOSPHATE
Phosphoglucomutase ↓
GLUCOSE-6-PHOSPHATE
Phosphohexomutase ↓
FRUCTOSE-6-PHOSPHATE
↓
2 PYRUVIC ACID
↓ **2 NADH + H^+** → **2 NAD^+**
2 LACTIC ACID

Main steps in anaerobic muscle glycolysis.

Under normal conditions, the hydrogens released during respiration by muscle cells are accepted by oxygen, which is the final hydrogen acceptor. During violent physical exercise, as in fast running, the supply of oxygen is insufficient to accept all the released hydrogens. Pyruvic acid itself becomes the hydrogen acceptor and is transformed into lactic acid. In this case, as noted before, only 3 molecules of ATP are produced instead of the 39 under aerobic conditions. Accumulation of lactic acid results in muscle fatigue, and the runner may get cramps. When the runner stops running, he pants for some time bringing oxygen to the muscles. In the presence of oxygen 1/5 of the lactic acid formed is metabolised to carbon dioxide and water, and energy is released as ATP. This energy is used in the re-synthesis of the remaining 4/5 of lactic acid to glycogen.

Kinds of Respiration

Hydrogen atoms removed during glucose metabolism are accepted by NAD^+, which is reduced to $NAD+H^+$. NAD^+ must be regenerated from $NADH+H^+$ in order to pick up more hydrogen atoms. If this did not happen glycosis would stop, resulting in the death of the organism. Living organisms have various mechanisms for disposing off hydrogen from $NADH+H^+$. The three main types of respiration are based on the manner in which organisms oxidise $NADH+H^+$ to NAD^+. In all these three types of respiration glycolysis (glucose to pyruvic acid) is the common feature. The fate of pyruvic acid and the method of hydrogen disposal determine the types of respiration, which are: (1) fermentation, (2) anaerobic respiration by some bacteria, and (3) aerobic respiration.

Fermentation takes place under anaerobic conditions and is of two main types, *alcoholic fermentation* and *atic acid fermentation (muscle glycolysis)*. *Alcoholic fermentation* is carried on by yeasts, some bacteria, and even green plants under lack of oxygen. Pyruvic acid is first decarboxylated to *acetaldehyde,* which is then reduced to *ethyl alcohol* by NADH, and NAD^+ is regenerated.

$$\text{Glucose} \xrightarrow{\text{Glycolysis}} \text{Pyruvic acid} \rightarrow \text{Acetaldehyde} \rightarrow \text{Ethyl alcohol.}$$

$$C_6H_{12}O_6 \qquad 2C_3H_4O_3 \qquad 2CH_3CHO \downarrow \qquad 2C_2H_5OH$$

$$NADH+H^+ \rightarrow NAD^+$$

Lactic acid fermentation (muscle glycolysis) is characteristic of animals and some forms of bacteria (e.g. latic acid bacteria). Pyruvic acid formed as a result of glycolysis acts as a hydrogen acceptor and yields *lactic acid.*

NAD^+ is regenerated. Both types of fermentation yield only two molecules of ATP.

$$\text{Glucose} \xrightarrow{\text{Glycolysis}} \text{Pyruvic acid} \xrightarrow[NADH+H^+ \rightarrow NAD^+]{} \text{Latic acid}$$

$$C_6H_{12}O_6 \qquad 2C_3H_4O_3$$

In anaerobic respiration of some bacteria, hydrogen is passed on to oxygen which is not in the free form. It is found as a part an in organic compound such as sulphate (SO_4^-) or nitrate (NO_3^-).

Aerobic respiration takes place in the presence of free oxygen. As usual, pyruvic acid is first formed from glucose by glycolysis. Pyruvic acid is completely oxidised through the Krebs citric acid cycle and the hydrogen transport system to yield carbon dioxide and water. Oxygen serves as the final hydrogen acceptor. For each molecule of glucose completely oxidised to carbon dioxide and water, 38 molecules of ATP are generated.

$$\text{Glucose} \xrightarrow{\text{Glycolysis}} 2\ \text{Pyruvic acid} \xrightarrow[\text{Hydrogen transport system}]{\text{Krebs cycle and}} CO_2 + H_2O.$$

Pathways in Intermediary Metabolism of Carbohydrate: The different pathways in the metabolism of carbohydrate are *glycogenolysis, glycolysis, Krebs citric acid cycle, gluconeogenesis* and the *pentose phosphate pathway* (Fig.).

Glycogenolysis: The breakdown of glycogen is called *glycogenolysis*. In the liver, the main end product of glycogen breakdown is *glucose*. In muscle the main products are *pyruvic acid* and *lactic acid*. Glycogen acts as a carbohydrate reserve. Whenever glucose is required, glycogen undergoes glycogenolysis, liberating glucose into the blood stream. The hormone *glucagon* stimulates the conversion of glycogen to glucose in the liver and thus causes a rise in blood sugar. Glucagon is secreted by the A-cells of the islets of Langerhans in the pancreas. *Epinephrine (adrenaline)* secreted by the medulla of the adrenal gland promotes conversion of glycogen to glucose in the liver and also conversion of glycogen to lactic acid in muscle during anaerobic metabolism.

Glycogenesis is the synthesis of *glycogen* (in animals) and *starch* (in plants) from glucose. When glucose is absorbed into the blood stream, some amount is immediately converted into glycogen in the liver. Some glucose passes from the liver into systemic circulation and is converted into glycogen in the muscles. An outline of glycogenesis is given below.

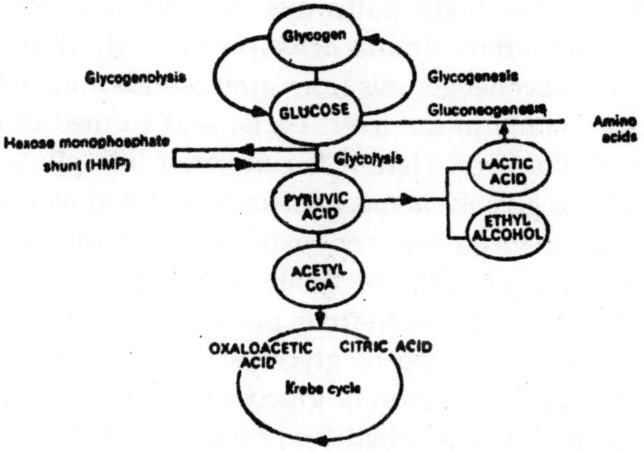

Pathways in intermediary carbohydrate metabolism.

Glucose is converted into *glucose-6-phosphate,* which is then converted into *glucose-1-phosphate.* Glucose-1-phosphate combines with *uridine triphosphate* (UTP) to form *uridine diphosphoglucose* (UDPG), with elimination of pyrophosphate (PPi).

Glucose -1- phosphate + UTP $\rightarrow$ UDP-glucose + pyrophosphate UDPG transfers the glucose molecule to the end of an existing glycogen chain. Repeated addition of one glucose unit at a time extends the glycogen chain.

UDP-glucose + Glycogen (n) $\rightarrow$ Glycogen (n + 1) + UDP. UDP can be reconverted to UTP by transfer of phospate from ATP. UDP+ATP $\rightleftharpoons$ UTP + ADP.

Glycolysis: The metabolic pathway starting with glucose and ending with pyruvic acid is called *glycolysis* (see Embden-Meyerhof-Parnas scheme).

Krebs citric acid cycle is the final common pathway of oxidation of carbohydrates, proteins and fats through acetyl-CoA, which is completely oxidised to carbon dioxide and water.

Gluconeogenesis is the formation of glucose or glycogen from non-carbohydrate precursors. The citric acid cycle and glycolysis are the main pathways of gluconeogenesis. The substrates are certain amino acids, lactic acid, glycerol and propionate. Gluconeogenesis from amino acids and lactic acid takes place mainly in the liver. Lactic acid formed in muscle is carried to the liver. Here it is converted into glucose by a reversal of the glycolysis mechanism and stored as glycogen. Pentose phosphate pathway or hexose monophosphate (HMP) shunt. In the liver, adipose tissue and lactating mammary glands, there is an alternative pathway to the Embden-Meyerhof-Parnas scheme of glycolysis and the Krebs citric acid cycle for the oxidation of glucose to carbon dioxide and water. This pathway is called the *pentose phosphate pathway* or *hexose monophosphate shunt*. In this pathway for every six glucose molecules in the beginning, five hexoses are regenerated while one glucose molecule is oxidised.

Metabolic Apparatus

The breakdown products of the three main classes of foods, carbohydrates, proteins and fats, can participate in glycolysis and the Krebs cycle. These product exist in 'metabolic pools' in the cytoplasm and can be utilised for cell respiration. Thus interconversion of proteins, carbohydrates and fats can occur through the glycolytic pathway and the Krebs cycle (Fig.). This metabolic interconversion is called the *metabolic mill*. Carbohydrates (polysaccharides) are hydrolysed during the process of digestion to form *monosaccharides*. Of these the hexose sugar *glucose* is the key compound in respiration. Other sugars like *galactose* and *fructose* can also serve as sources of energy, and are readily convertible into glucose. *Glycogen* can also be converted into glucose. Glucose is metabolised through the glycolytic pathway and Krebs cycle to yield energy in the form of ATP.

Proteins are digested into their constituent amino acids.

These amino acids undergo *deamination* and enter at various points in the glycolytic pathway and the Krebs cycle. During deamination the amino (—NH_2) group of the amino acid is removed. Thus *alanine* on deamination forms *oxaloacetic* acid, and *glutamic acid* forms α *-ketoglutaric acid*. The amino acids alanine, serine, cysteine, cystine, glycine, threonine, hydroxyproline, valine and methionine enter the glycolytic pathway at the *pyruvic acid* stage. Aspartic acid is converted into *oxaloacetic acid* and enters the Krebs cycle. Methionine, leucine, isoleucine and valine enter the Krebs cycle at the *succinyl CoA* stage.

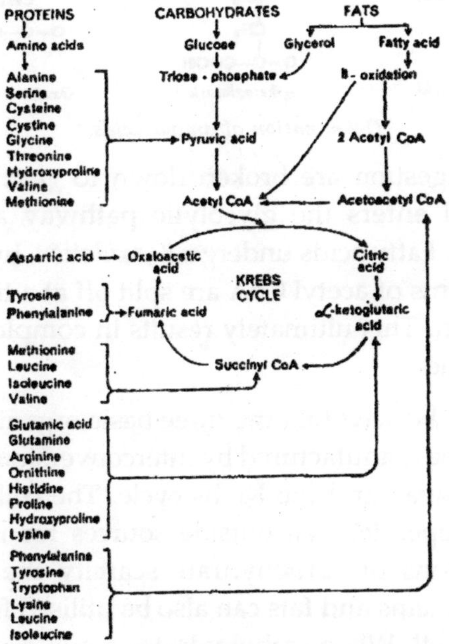

The metabolic mill.

Glutamic acid, glutamine, arginine, ornithine, histidine, proline, hydroxyproline and lysine enter the Krebs cycle at the, α *-ketoglutaric acid* stage. Phenylalanine, tyrosine, tryptophan, lysine, leucine and isoleucine enter as *acetoacetyl CoA.* The pathway can be reversed under certain conditions. Thus by addition of an amino ($—NH_2$) group *(amination)* α -ketoglutaric acid forms *glutamic acid.* Such amino acids which are synthesised by the cell are called *non-essential amino acids.* They are formed by the cell itself and need not be taken in the food. On the other hand amino acids which are not synthesised by the cell, but must be obtained from food are called *essential amino acids.*

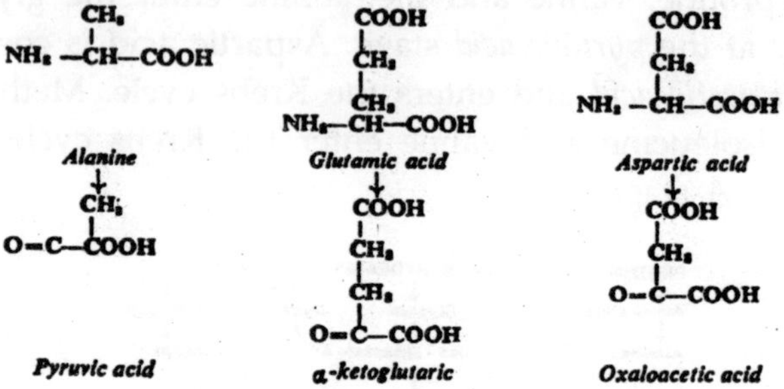

Deamination of amino acids.

Fats on digestion are broken down to *glycerol* and *fatty acids.* Glycerol enters the glycolytic pathway at the *triose-phosphate stage.* Fatty acids undergo β *-oxidation,* by which two-carbon fragments of acetyl CoA are split off at a time from the fatty acid chain. This ultimately results in complete oxidation of the fatty acid.

It will thus be seen that the three basic organic substances of the cell can be manufactured by interconversion through the glycolytic pathway and the Krebs cycle. The cell is therefore not entirely dependent on outside sources for its materials. Under conditions of carbohydrate scarcity the breakdown products of proteins and fats can also be utilised for providing energy to the cell. When carbohydrates are in excess, fats can be synthesised from them. Thus eating of excess of potatoes (carbohydrate) results in fatness. Conversely, after prolonged fasting a person becomes thin, as his fat reserves are utilised for cell respiration. This permits a degree of flexibility in the biochemical system of the cell.

5

Various Metabolisms

Genes control various traits in an organism through a control exercised on the developmental processes. Such a control is due to synthesis of proteins, which is under direct control of genes. Some of these proteins synthesised by genes are enzymes and control biosynthetic pathways.

That genes express themselves through synthesis of enzymes was demonstrated for the first time in 1941 by G.W. Beadle and E.L. Tatum (both Noble Prize winners of 1958), due to their discovery of biochemical mutations in *Neurospora*.

Based on their work, Beadle and Tatum proposed a concept called one gene-one enzyme hypothesis. Such a hypothesis means that if in a biosynthetic pathway several steps are involved, each step is controlled by a specific enzyme, which is synthesised under the control of a specific gene (Fig.).

Mutations in these genes helped in elucidating several biosynthetic pathways in a variety of organisms, particularly in microbes like fungi and bacteria.

This will be illustrated with the help of some examples in this chapter. For the study of these biochemical mutations, and mutations for resistance against phages and antibiotics, microbial systems have proved to be particularly useful. Large populations can be handled in these microbes, so that even rare recombinants and mutations, with very low frequencies, can be easily detected.

This has given rise to an area of study in genetics, popularly described as 'microbial genetics', which may also include biochemical genetics. Cases of mutations for resistance against phages and antibiotics in bacteria will also be described briefly in this chapter.

gene A	gene B	gene C
↓	↓	↓
enzyme a	enzyme b	enzyme c
↓	↓	↓
precursor. → product A	→	product B → product C
(step a)	(step b)	(step c)

Diagrammatic representation of the biosynthesis of a product C involving three steps.

Elementary Errors of Metabolism

Earliest cases of biochemical mutations were described in man by A.E. Garrod in 1909 in his book *"Inborn Errors of Metabolism"*. There are three important diseases associated with metabolic breakdown of phenylalamine (Fig.).

(i) Phenylketonuria is due to accumulation of phenylpyruvic acid and causes mental disorders. Children suffering with this disease are known as *phenylpyruvic idiots* and are unable to breakdown *phenylpyruvic acid* into hydroxy-phenylpyruvic acid,

(ii) Alcaptonuria is due to lack of ability to breakdown *homogentisic acid* into *acetoacetic acid.*

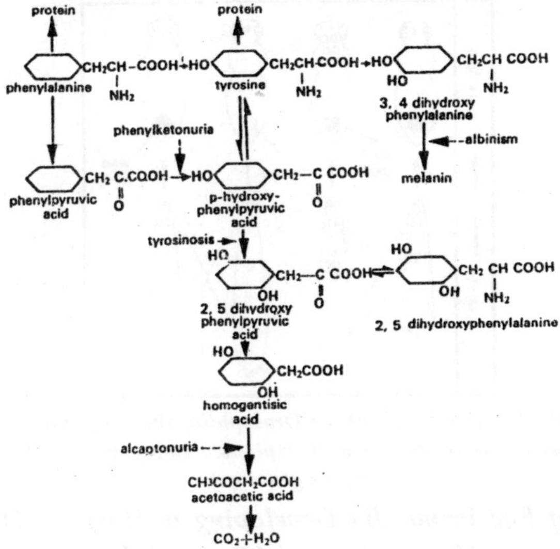

Biochemistry of degradation of phenylalanine.

Due to accumulation of homogentisic acid, the urine of patients suffering with this disease turns black as soon as it comes in contact with air.

(iii) Albinism is due to absence of melanin pigment and individuals suffering with this disease are incapable of converting *dihydroxy-phenylalanine* into *melanin.* Another disease tyrosinosis is also associated with the same metabolic pathway (Fig.).

Eye Transplantation: Before having initiated his work on *Neurospora,* G.W. Beadle had conducted eye transplantation experiments in *Drosophila* in collaboration with B. Ephrussi in Europe. It is due to the frustration he had with this work, that he subsequently shifted to *Neurospora.*

Beadle and Ephrussi transplanted larval embryonic eye primordia from one mutant type into another and studied the development of pigment in such transplanted eyes. The results of these transplantation experiments are presented in Figure and Table.

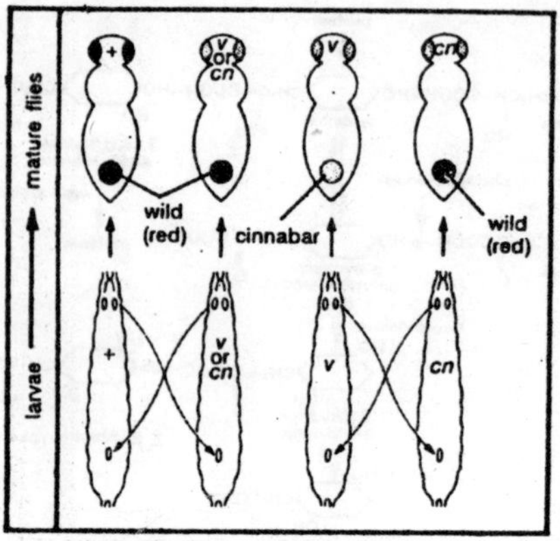

Eye transplantation experiments in Drosophila, showing autonomous and non-autonomous development of implanted embryonic eye discs into various genotypes.

Colour of Eye Primordia Developing in Hosls of Different Mutant Types in Drosophila.

Host eye colour	*Donor eye colour*	*Transplanted eye colour*
Wild	Vermilion	Wild
Vermilion	Wild	Wild
Wild	Cinnabar	Wild
Cinnabar	Wild	Wild
Cinnabar	Vermilion	Wild
Vermilion	Cinnabar	Cinnabar

It can be noticed in Table that, when wild type eyes are transplanted on a vermilion or cinnabar host, wild type eyes develop, indicating that phenotype of eyes in this case is independent of host. In reciprocal transplantations, when vermilion or cinnabar eyes are transplanted on wild type, these transplanted eyes also develop into wild type, because a diffusible substance (probably an enzyme) from host helps the transplanted eyes to develop into wild type.

Crucial results were obtained when reciprocal transplantations were made between vermilion and cinnabar. When vermilion eye is transplanted on cinnabar, a wild type eye develops, indicating that a diffusible substance from cinnabar enables the transplanted vermilion eye to develop into wild type. However, when cinnabar eye is transplanted on vermilion, no diffusible substance is available which would enable cinnabar to develop into wild type.

This indicated that vermilion colour appears due to a block appearing earlier in biosynthetic pathway than in case of cinnabar. The suggested biosynthetic pathway is shown in Figure.

Biochemical Mutations in Neurospora: Life cycle of *Neurospora,* a member of Ascomycetes. This organism was extensively utilised in the study of biochemical mutations initially by Beadle and Tatum and subsequently by other workers. It can be grown on a culture medium which contains a few simple salts, some sugar and biotin. From these raw materials, the organism is capable of manufacturing all other compounds required for its growth.

As a result of mutations, strains may be obtained which lack the ability to synthesise one or more of these compounds. While the wild strain which is capable of growing on *minimal medium* is known as prototroph, the nutritionally deficient mutants are known as auxotrophs.

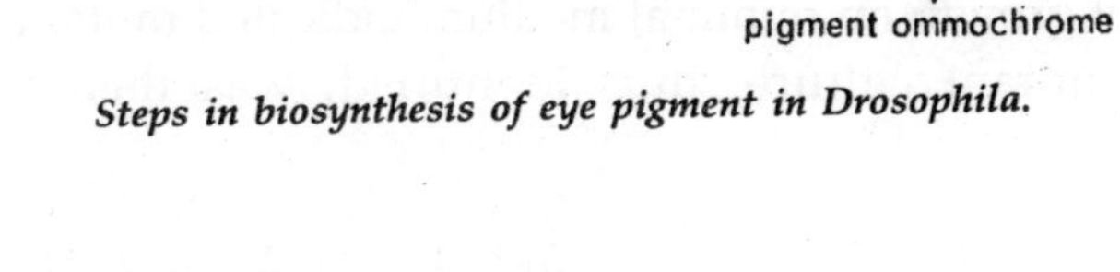

Steps in biosynthesis of eye pigment in Drosophila.

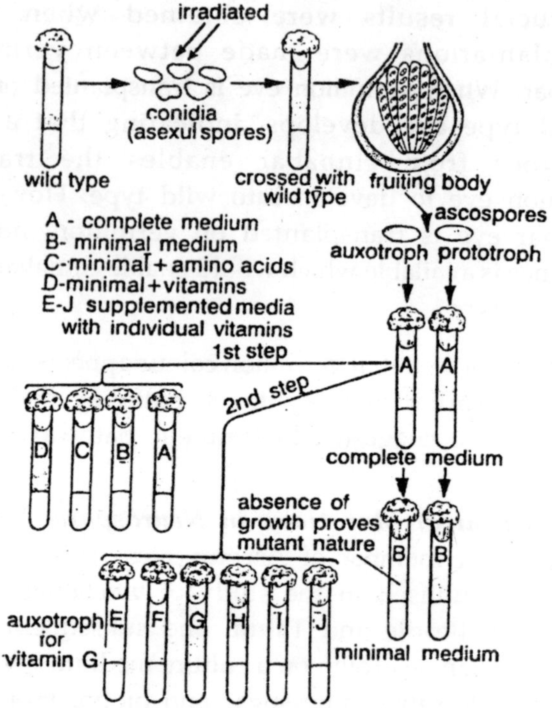

Detection of biochemical mutations in Neurospora.

Method of Total Separation

Beadle and Tatum irradiated conidia of *Neurospora,* mated these irradiated conidia with wild type and subsequently studied segregation for induced mutations, if any. One of the advantages of using *Neurospora* is that the four products of meiosis stay in same ascus and segregation can be easily studied in eight ascospores of an ascus. For the study of segregation, individual ascospores were first grown on complete medium (a medium having all metabolites in addition to minimal medium), so that both mutant and wild types may grow.

These were then transferred to minimal medium. Lack of growth on minimal medium indicated mutant nature. Each mutant culture, thus identified, was then tried on supplemented media (media, containing each specific metabolite in addition to minimal medium) and specific nutritional requirement, for which mutation had occurred, was thus identified (Fig.).

This technique originally utilised by Beadle and Tatum, called 'total isolation method' though provided most reliable data, but was very laborious, since individual ascospores had to be tested. Therefore, various modifications were subsequently used by different workers.

Replica Plating Method

One popular modified technique is known as *replica plating technique,* suggested by J. Lederberg in 1952. This technique can be conveniently utilised not only in *Neurospora,* but also in other microorganisms forming colonies.

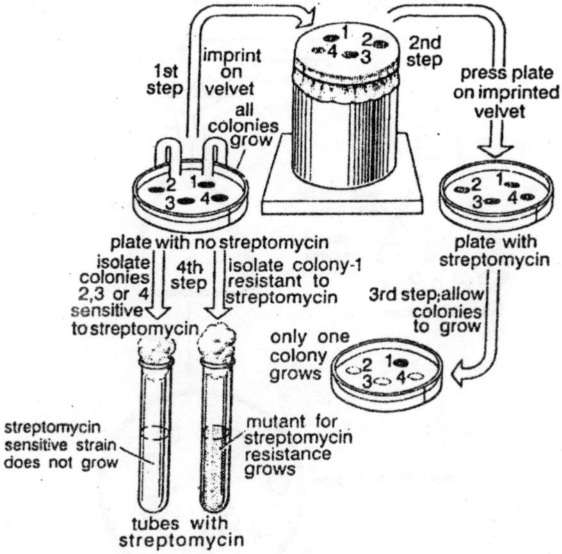

Replica plating technique for detection and isolation of mutations in microorganisms.

The material (ascospores or spores) is first grown on complete medium. For instance, if streptomycin resistant mutants are to be isolated, material should be allowed to grow on medium lacking streptomycin, so that both mutant and wild types may grow.

These colonies are imprinted on velveteen by inverting the petri plate, so that all the colonies are imprinted and leave spores at corresponding positions on velveteen. This will then be the master pattern and other plates having streptomycin can then be pressed on velveteen to get an impression. On this plate now, only mutants for streptomycin resistance will grow. Knowing the position of a mutant colony, corresponding colony in original plate without streptomycin can be marked and used for isolation and multiplication of the mutant. *Replica plating technique,* involving four different steps, is illustrated in Figure.

Filtration Enrichment Technique: Concentration of auxotrophs (nutritional mutants) can also be increased by

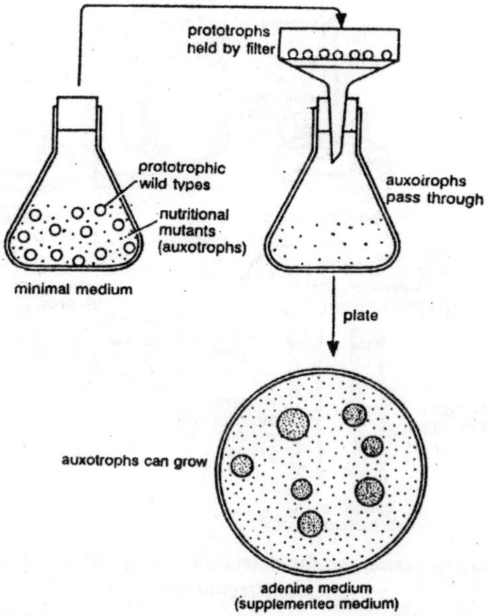

The filtration enrichment method for selecting forward mutations giving auxotrophs.

filtration of a culture grown in suspension culture with minimal medium on which only prototrophs will grow. During filtration, due to filamentous growth of fungi, the prototrophs will be filtered out and only non-growing auxotrophic mutant spores will be available in filtrate, which can be subjected to usual method of isolation and testing (Fig.). The filtration method was described by Woodward in 1954 and is known as *Woodward's filtration technique.*

System of Penicillin Enrichment

Bacteria and fungi like *Neurospora,* in proliferating stage, is sensitive to penicillin. Therefore, in a suspension culture with minimal medium, if penicillin is added, the prototrophs (being capable of growing in the minimal medium) will be killed. The auxotrophs will survive due to lack of growth. After killing prototrophs thus, the penicillin can be removed by washing the cells on a filter. If the culture is now plated on a solid medium supplemented with a specific chemical, auxotrophs deficient in this chemical will grow and can be counted and isolated for further study.

Mutations in E. coli for Resistance against Phages or Antibiotics: Mutations for resistance can be isolated by spreading large population of bacteria (10^9 cells) on a plate containing thick layer of phage (*e.g.*, T_1) or an antibiotic as the case may be. The surviving colonies would be resistant and represent mutants. S. Luria and M. Delbruck (in 1943) conducted experiments to find the origin of these mutants. There were two possibilities:

(i) these could be random genetic changes or

(ii) these could arise as physiological adaptation to the presence of phage or antibiotic.

In order to test, which of these two alternatives was correct, Luria and Delbruck allowed growth of *E. coli* cells (using 10^3 cells per ml) in two sets:

(i) 20 tubes each with 0.2 ml of medium, and

(ii) one tube with 10 ml of medium.

After an incubation period, each of the 20 tubes (0.2 ml) were spread on plates with a layer of phage (or antibiotic). Similarly ten 0.2 ml samples from 10 ml tube in (ii) above were drawn and plated on 10 plates. It was shown that individual 0.2 ml cultures showed large variation, while samples drawn from 10 ml bulk culture did not show any variation in the frequency of resistant colonies. The variation in 0.2 ml culture was mainly due to differences in the time of appearance of mutation during multiplication. The experiment proved that mutations appeared as random genetic changes and not as physiological adaptation, because if the latter was true, no variation in mutation frequency in 0.2 ml tubes should be expected.

Interrupting Cell Counting

In mutation studies, since a known number of cells need to be plated for calculating mutation rates, it is necessary to count cells per unit volume (per ml). This can be achieved by any of the following methods:

(i) A hemocytometer may be placed under the microscope and the cells may be counted on a marked grid,

(ii) A calibration curve using different levels of turbidity (with known counts of cells) can be drawn (turbidity measured as light passing through the suspension). Then for samples with unknown counts, turbidity may be measured and corresponding counts may be determined from turbidity curve,

(iii) Suspensions of known dilution are plated on solid medium and colonies are counted (each colony derived from a single cell),

(iv) Electronic cell counters may be used.

Calculation of Mutation Rates and Frequencies: Students of cell biology should recognise, that mutation rate and mutation frequency are two different parameter to study the occurrence of mutations. In the experiment of Luria and Delbruck described earlier, 20 culture tubes (0.2 ml) were used for study of mutations for resistance against T_1 phage. In this case 11 out of 21 tubes had no mutant cells. If frequencies of culture tubes showing 1, 2, 3, ... 100 (or more) mutant colonies are worked out, they exhibit a Poisson distribution (mean frequency of class with no mutations = 11/20).

In Figure, it can be seen that when we start with one cell, the total number of cell divisions at the end = n-1 (n= number of cells at the end). Therefore, if n is very high (10^8 per ml) relative to very small original number, then n gives a sufficiently accurate estimate of cell divisions. Now, if mutation rate per cell division is assumed to be μ, mutation events per tube will be $\mu \times n = \mu n$. According to Poisson distribution

$$f_{(0)} = e^{-m} = e^{-\mu n}$$

Therefore, $f_0 = 11/20 = .0.55 = e^{-\mu^{(0.2\times10^8)}}$, which gives $\mu = 3 \times 10^{-8}$ mutations per cell division. Mutation frequency per cell, on the other hand is calculated as (mutants in all 20 tubes)/ $(20 \times 0.2 \times 10^8)$, which was found to be 5.7×10^{-7} per cell.

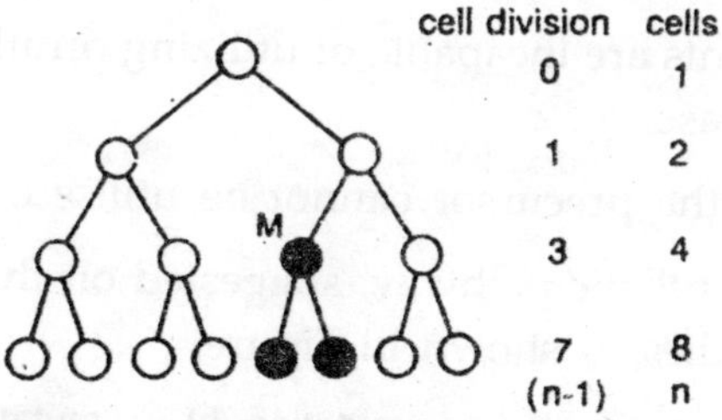

A simple cell pedigree showing a mutation at M.

Biochemical Mutations and Biosynthetic Pathways: As shown earlier in case of synthesis of eye pigment in *Drosophila*, a biosynthetic pathway can be worked out using biochemical mutations, since mutation in a particular gene leads to block in a particular step of biosynthetic pathway.

The step which has been blocked can be known either by accumulation of an intermediate product or by recovery of trait due to supply of another intermediate product. This will be illustrated by two additional examples.

Arginine Combination

In *Neurospora,* following three kinds of mutations for arginine synthesis were isolated.

(1) Mutations, which grow only when arginine is supplied and do not grow with the help of either ornithine or citrulline alone.

(2) Mutations, which grow only when either citrulline or arginine is supplied, but do not grow when only ornithine is supplied.

(3) Mutations which can grow only, when either ornithine or citrulline or arginine is supplied.

These mutants indicate that, in the first case:

(i) mutants are incapable of utilizing ornithine or citrulline; in the second case,

(ii) mutants are incapable of utilizing ornithine; but in the last case,

(iii) only the precursor cannot be utilised.

The biosynthetic pathway, suggested on the basis of these mutation studies, is shown in Figure.

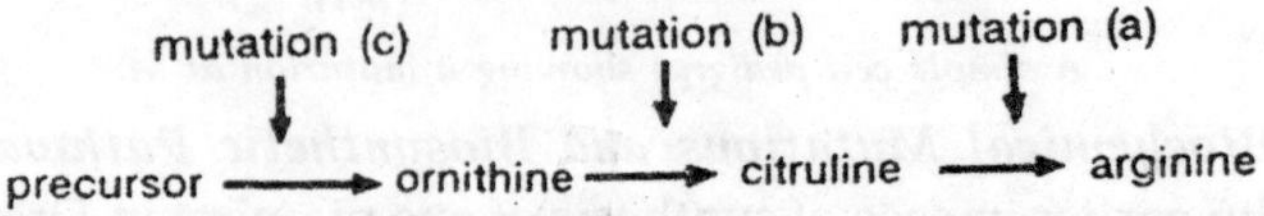

Different steps in the synthesis of arginine and three different mutations blocking three steps.

Synthesis of Tryptophan in Bacteria and Neurospora

Salmonella Typhimurium: In *Salmonella typhimurium,* four kinds of mutants for tryptophan synthesis could be isolated. These mutations are listed in Table and include the following:

(i) *trp-8* does not have the ability to synthesise anthranilic acid but the growth can be restored by addition of either of the following compounds—anthranilic acid, indole glycerol phosphate, indole or tryptophan.

(ii) *trp*-2 and *trp*-4 can not grow on either the minimal medium or on the supplemented medium with anthranilic acid, but can grow on addition of either indole glycerol phosphate, or indole or tryptophan.

(iii) *trp*-3 can grow only on a supplemented medium with either indole or tryptophan, but not on any other medium,

Different Mutants and their Response to Different Growth Media in Salmonella Typhimurium.

Gene mutation	Growth response					Accumulated product
	Minimal medium	Supplemented media*				
		Ant	IGP	I	T	
trp-8	–	+	+	+	+	—
trp-2,-4	–	–	+	+	+	Ant
trp-3	–	–	–	+	+	IGP
trp-1,-6,-7,-9,-10,-11	–	–	–	–	+	IGP & I

* Ant = anthranilic acid; IGP = indole glycerol phosphate; I = indole; T = tryptophan. + sign indicates growth ; – sign indicates lack of growth.

(iv) *trp-1, 6, 7, 9, 10, 11,* etc. can grow only on a supplemented medium with tryptophan and on no other medium.

These different mutants indicate interruption of biochemical pathway at different steps.

Escherichia Coli: In Escherichia coli also five different kinds of mutations called *trp*A, *trp*B, *trp*C, *trp*D and *trp*E were identified. These mutations are similar to those described for Salmonella, and shown in Figure and Table. The traced out using the mutants described above for Salmonella typhimurium and Escherichia coli.

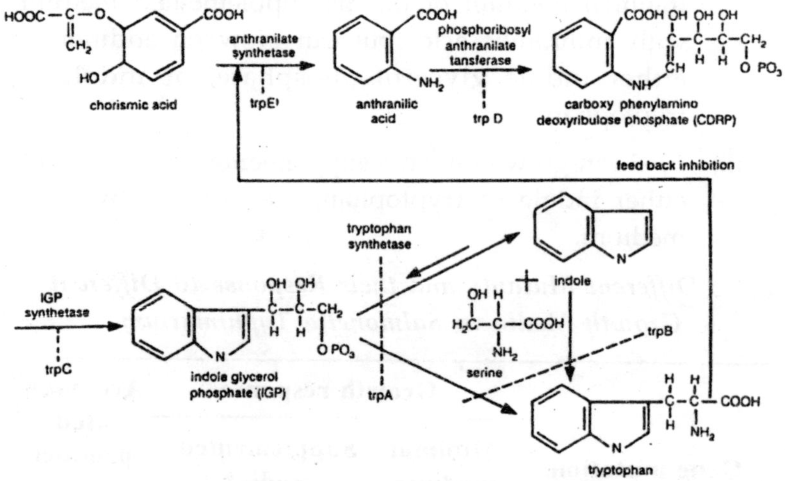

Deterrent steps in the synthesis of amino acid tryptophan, showing the enzymes and genes for each step.

Tryptophan Synthetase in Neurospora and Bacteria: It has been shown that the last two steps of tryptophan metabolism in Neurospora as well as in bacteria are controlled by the same enzyme tryptophan synthetase, so that even mutants lacking the ability to utilise indole do not have *tryptophan synthetase* enzyme. In *Neurospora,* this enzyme consists of only one component. But in *E. coli* and *Salmonella,* it has two components:

(i) 'A' component affecting penultimate step in Figure, so

that *trpA* mutants lacking A component can be supplemented by both indole and tryptophan and

(ii) 'B' component, which affects last step in Figure. So that *trpB* mutants lacking B component must be supplemented directly with tryptophan.

It has also been shown that in mutants for this enzyme, protein is synthesised, but it is unable to perform enzymatic function.

The presence of two components (A and B) of tryptophan synthetase enzyme, synthesised under the control of two different genes suggests that a particular enzyme may consist of more than one polypeptides, each synthesised under the control of a different functional unit called cistron. Therefore, it was suggested that the concept of one gene-one enzyme proposed initially by Beadle and Tatum should be modified into one cistron-one polypeptide hypothesis.

Linear order of Genes in genome and that of Enzymes in a Biosynthetic Pathway: In this chapter, earlier we have shown that each step of a biosynthetic pathway is controlled by a specific enzyme synthesised under the influence of a specific gene. In several cases, although not universally it has been shown that the genes involved in different steps of a biosynthetic pathway are clustered and found on the genetic map in the same linear order in which their corresponding enzymes are used in the biosynthetic pathway. This will be illustrated with the help of two examples.

Tryptophan Metabolism: It has been earlier shown that for tryptophan synthesis in *Salmonella,* five enzymes are needed for five steps earlier described as 1, 2, 3, 4, 5. It was found that the genes for three enzymes in *Salmonella* are found in the same order in which the steps are found in the biosynthetic pathway.

Histidine Metabolism: More than 500 mutations for

histidine metabolism in *Salmonella* were mapped. These were linked in nine closely linked loci A to H, each affecting a different enzyme in the synthesis of histidine. The linear order of genes in the genome was found to follow largely the order of steps of a metabolic pathway, in which the products of these genes are utilised.

For several other traits including proline, threonine and isoleucine—valine metabolism in *Salmonella,* a similar clustering of genes was observed. This suggests, that at a primitive stage, biochemical synthesis during evolution must have first organised on the chromosome itself.

6

The Ultrastructure

In 1880, Kalliker for the first time recognised the structures now known as mitochondria. However, the credit for the discovery of mitochondria is given to W. Flemming and R. Altaian. While Flemming described some thread-like structures in 1882, Airman described granules in 1890. These cell inclusions were later called mitochondria (mitos=thread, chondrion=granule) by C. Benda in 1897. These evidences for the presence of mitochondria were available only in the animal cells. The first evidence for the presence of mitochondria in plant cells *(Nymphaea)* was given by F. Meves in 1904. Since then, mitochondria have been shown in all kinds of plant and animal cells. However, an important advancement in the study of mitochondria was made with the isolation of liver mitochondria for the first time by Bensley and Hoerr in 1934. The mitochondria of a cell are collectively designated as chondriome.

Morphology: The mitochondria can be more easily examined in cultured cells rather than under *in vivo* condition (living organisms). They can be conveniently studied with the help of a phase contrast microscope. To facilitate further examination, the mitochondria may be stained with Janus green which stains the organelle with a greenish blue stain due to oxidation of dye by cytochrome oxidase. In cell extracts, due to differential centrifugation, mitochondria sediment at 5000 to 24000g, while in living cells by ultracentrifugation (200,000 to 400,000g), mitochondria are deposited intact at the centrifugal pole.

In a light microscope, the mitochondria appear as rod-shaped, filamentous or granular structures in majority of the cells. They appear as granular in spermatozoa and oocytes and club-shaped in liver cells. The morphology of mitochondria varies not only from one cell to another, but also within the same cell (Fig.). Depending upon certain functions also, they

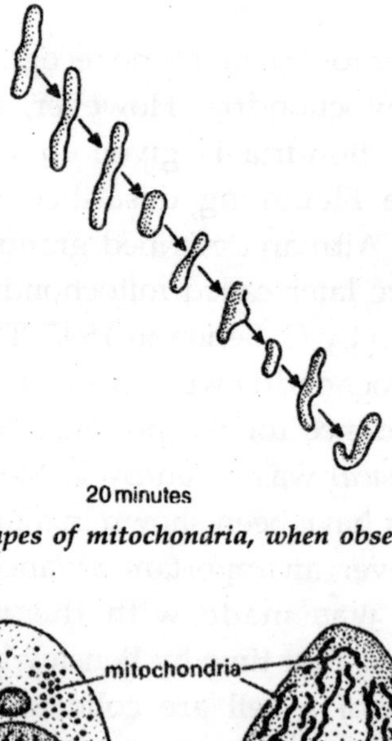

Rapid changes in shapes of mitochondria, when observed in a living cell.

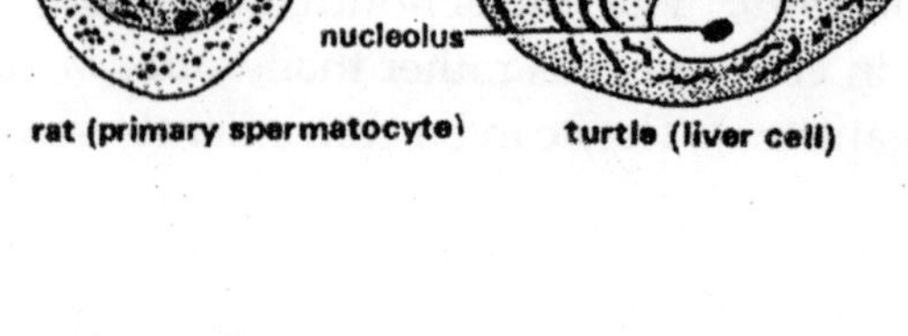

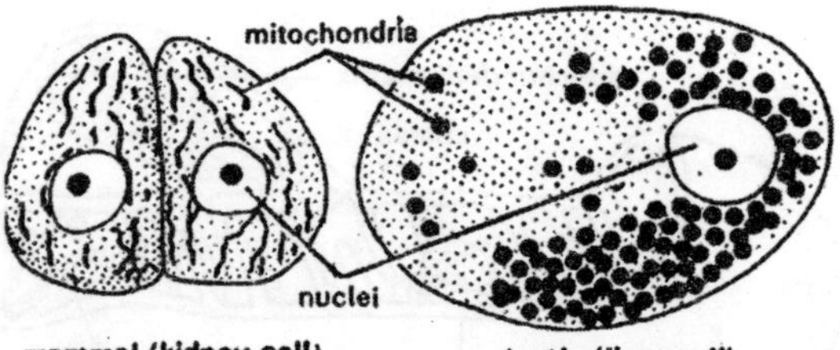

Cells of different materials showing size differences in mitochondria (redrawn from Swanson: Cytology and Cytogenetics, 1957).

may change their shape and may take the shape of a club or a tennis racket. The mitochondria normally vary in size from 0.5 μ A to 2.0 μ (Fig.) and are therefore not easy to detect in light microscope. However, their length may sometimes reach upto 7.0 μ. The number of mitochondria per cell varies according to the function and volume of cells. There may be 50-5000 mitochondira in a cell. The number may reach upto 500,000 in some kind of protozoa. Rarely mitochondria may also be branched.

The Mitochondria

In most of the cells, mitochondria in electron micrographs show a quite smooth outer membrane about 6nm thick. Inside and separated from the outer membrane by a space is present the inner membrane also 6nm thick. Therefore, a mitochondrion has a double membrane envelope, the two membranes being separated by a space 6-8 nm. The inner membrane is not smooth and forms mitochondrial crests. This inner membrane divides the mitochondria into two chambers, namely (i) peri-mitochondrial space between outer membrane and inner membrane which is continuous into the core of the crests, and (ii) the inner chamber inside the inner membrane, which is occupied by a relatively dense material called the mitochondrial matrix. The matrix is generally homogeneous, but may rarely show finely filamentous or fibrous structures.

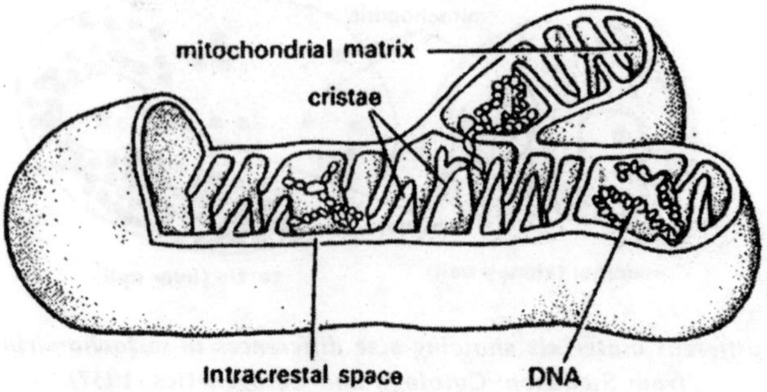

A single mitochondrion showing cristae and DNA.

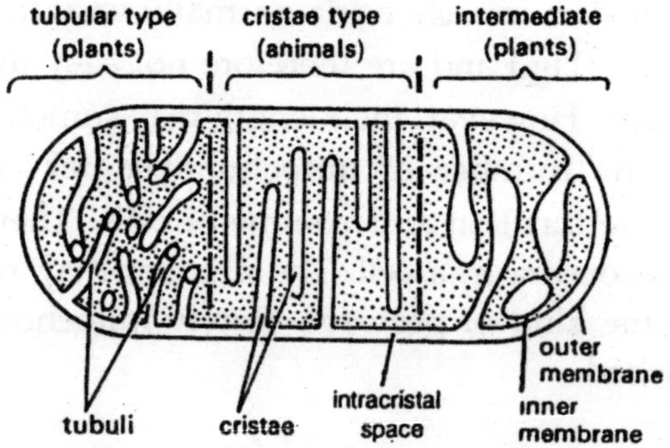

A sectional view of different kinds of mitochondria.

The detailed structure of mitochondrion is shown in Figure. As can be seen, the inner membrane is convoluted, the folds consisting of double membranes and called cristae (animals). These infoldings are tubular in plants and are known as tubuli or microvilli. Frequently in plants, an intermediate type of infoldings shown in Figure are also found.

The fine structure of a mitochondrion can change in different cells of a tissue, at different stages of development or in different physiological and pathological conditions. This suggests that mitochondrial membranes are dynamic structures. The cristae may be simple or branched forming a complex network which provides access to the respiratory enzymes and also provides additional membrane surface.

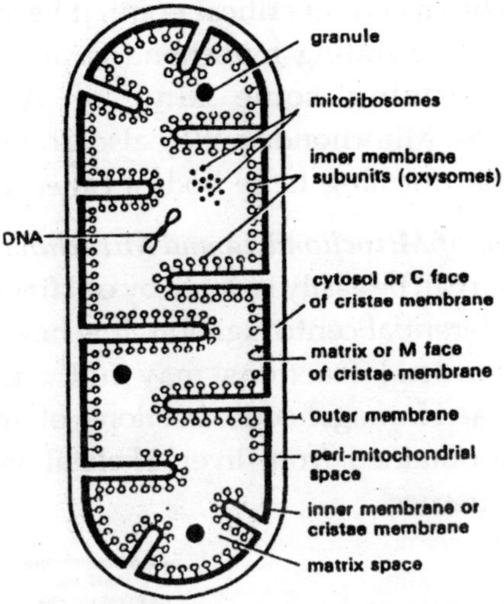

A mitochondrion in sectional view, showing oxysomes.

Attached to M face (facing matrix) of inner membrane are repeated units of stalked particles called elementary particles, inner membrane subunits or oxysomes (Fig.). These particles are approximately 8.5 nm (85°A) in diameter. These so called 'elementary particles' (also called as 'F_1 particles') are regularly spaced at intervals of 10 nm on the inner surface of these membranes. According to some estimates, there are 10^4 to 10^5 elementary particles per mitochondrion. When the mitochondrial cristae are disrupted by sonic vibrations, submitochondrial particles (sonic particles) are obtained and oxysomes are seen attached on their outer surface. These submitochondrial particles are responsible for respiratory chain phosphorylation. However, in the absence of oxysomes, the particles lose their capacity of phosphorylation as shown by dissolution and reconstitution of these particles (Fig.). The oxysomes have been identified as molecules of ATPase enzyme (coupling factor F_1) responsible for catalyzing the terminal step of ATP synthesis.

The mitochondria may be altered due to action of various agents, but most of these changes are reversible. Only if the change reaches a certain critical point, it becomes irreversible. Sometimes degenerating mitochondria are seen at places of autolysis, forming some kind of lysosomes called cytolysosomes. Mitochondria may also undergo degeneration due to fusion, forming large bodies called chondriospheres.

Isolation of Mitochondria and Mitochondrial Membranes: Mitochondria can be easily isolated by cell fractionation brought about by differential centrifugation. It is however, known that the mitochondrial fractions may not entirely consist of mitochondria. Homogeneous fractions of mitochondria can however be obtained from liver, skeletal muscle, heart and some other tissues.

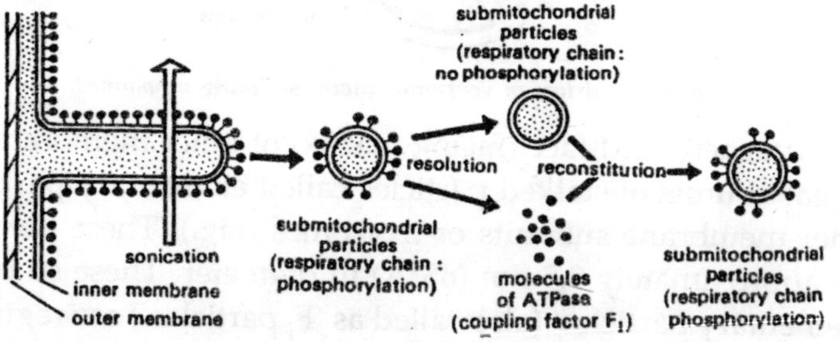

A diagrammatic representation showing the role of oxysomes in submitochondrial particles.

In recent years, two mitochondrial membranes could also be separated by density gradient centrifugation. The outer membrane can be separated by causing a swelling which can be brought about by breakage followed by contraction of inner membrane and matrix. Two detergents, namely 'digitonin' and 'lubrol' are often used for this purpose. Since outer membrane is lighter, much stronger centrifugal force is needed to separate it. In a gradient centrifugation for the same reason, a less dense gradient will be required. When outer membrane is removed with digitonin, a so-called mitoplast which includes inner membrane and matrix can be obtained. The mitoplast has pseudopodia and can carry out oxidative phosphorylation.

Such a separation of two membranes has enabled localisation of mitochondrial enzyme systems.

Chemical Format

Chemically, mitochondria mainly consist of proteins (65-70%) and lipids (25-30%). These two classes of compounds will constitute about 90-99% of the organelle. However, a small part of RNA and DNA is also known to be present. The presence of DNA has been demonstrated by techniques like autoradiography, enzyme hydrolysis and electron microscopy (less than 1% of cellular DNA in *Neurospora* is found in mitochondria). Mitochondria thus have their own DNA, tRNA (transfer RNA), RNA polymerase, ribosomes (mitoribosomes), amino acid-activating enzymes, etc. The mitochondrial DNA differs from nuclear DNA and resembles bacterial DNA. It is ring shaped in animals and linear in plants except in yeast. This DNA has been shown to be unrelated to nuclear DNA and is associated with extrachromosomal mitochondrial inheritance. Therefore, mitochondria have their separate protein synthesizing machinery which is independent of nuclear control. Mitochondria are, therefore, considered as semi-autonomous. The possibility of their origin from the nuclear envelope through promitochondrial stage has been suggested and cannot be ruled out.

The outer membrane fraction has a 40% lipid content, while inner membrane has only 20% lipid content. The outer membrane also contains more cholesterol and phosphatidyl inositol, though content of cardiolipin is low. It shows that lipid/protein ratio in the inner membrane is relatively low suggesting that intercalation of protein in the inner membrane is of a higher order, a fact which has been confirmed by electron microscopy.

A variety of vitamins and enzyme systems have been observed in mitochondria. A list of enzymes found in different mitochondrial fractions, is presented in Table.

Enzyme Distribution in Mitochondria

1. Outer membrane
   Monoamine oxidase
   NADH-cytochrome C reductase
   Kynurenine hydroxylase Fatty acid CoA ligase

2. Peri-mitochondrial space
   Adenylate kinase
   Nucleoside diphosphokinase

3. Inner membrane
   Respiratory chain enzymes & coenzymes
   — NADH dehydrogenase complex (NAD)
   — Flavin adenine dinucleotide (FAD)
   — Diphosphopyridine nucleotide (DPN)
   — Cytochrome b-c, complex
   (Cyt a & Cyt b, Cyt c, Cyt a_3, Cyt c_1,)
   — Cytochrome oxidase complex
   — Ubiquinone or coenyme Q
   ATP synthase, F_0F_1ATPase
   Succinate dehydrogenase
   β-hydroxy butyrate dehydrogenase
   Carnitine fatty acid acyl transferase

4. Matrix
   Pyruvate dehydrogenase complex
   Enzymes of TCA cycle
   Malate and isocitrate dehydrogenases
   Fumarase and aconitase
   Citrate synthetase
   — Keto acid dehydrogenases
   — Oxidation enzymes

As can be seen in Table, different components of respiratory chain phosphorylation are found in cristae, *i.e.* in the inner membrane. These enzyme systems associated with cristae include a number of dehydrogenases and cytochromes. The locations of these components are shown in Fig. and their roles in respiration.

Genome in Mitochondria

Remarkable variation has been observed in the size of mitochondrial genome (mtDNA), which varies from 6kb (*Plasmodium*) to 36kb (*Arabidopsis*). The mtDNA can be circular or linear in shape (linear mtDNA has been found in many ciliates, protozoa, algae, slime molds and oomycetous fungi). The entire nucleotide sequence of mtDNA in as many as~50 species of animals and plants are now available throwing new light on the origin of mitochondria from bacteria .

The gene content in mtDNA is relatively low, when compared with that of cpDNA (chloroplast DNA) in green plants. The number of genes in mtDNA varies from 5 in *Plasmodium* to 94 in *Reclinomonas* (number of genes in cpDNA is generally more than 100). The four genes that are common to all mtDNAs are *cob, coxl,* and the two genes for ribosomal RNA *(rns* and *rnl).*

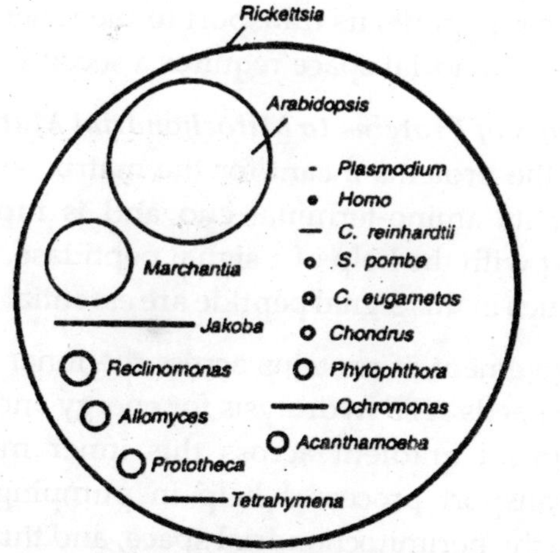

A cristae membrane showing the distribution of different dehydrogenases and cytochromes on M face and C face.

Transport of Proteins into Mitochondria: The mitochondrion contains a distinct set of proteins, but only a few of these proteins are encoded by mitochondrial genome. The proteins encoded by the mitochondrial genome (mtDNA) generally form only some subunits of protein complexes meant for the inner membrane of mitochondria, the other subunits being encoded by the nuclear genome and later transported to mitochondria. Therefore, major proportion of proteins (or their subunits) in the mitochondrion are synthesised in the cytoplasm outside the mitochondria and are later transported to the mitochondrion. Special mechanisms are needed for this transport of proteins and will be briefly discussed.

The precursors of mitochondrial proteins are synthesised in the cytoplasm and after their release from polyribosomes into the cytosol they are taken up by the mitochondria within a minute or two. These proteins may belong to either the outer membrane, or the inner membrane, or the perimitochondrial space or the mitochondrial matrix and the mechanism of transport may differ in each case. While the transport of a protein to outer membrane or to mitochondrial matrix requires a single signal peptide, its transport to the inner membrane or the peri-mitochondrial space requires a second signal peptide.

Transport of Proteins to Mitochondrial Matrix: The signal peptide in the proteins meant for the matrix consists of 20-80 residues at its amino-terminal end and is rapidly removed after import with the help of a signal peptidase. Only 12 of the 20-50 residues in this signal peptide are essential for the import.

The movement of proteins across the inner mitochondrial membrane needs ATP hydrolysis for energy and also needs an electrochemical gradient across this inner membrane. The electron transport processes help in pumping H^+ from the matrix into the perimitochondrial space, and thus maintain the electrochemical gradient necessary for protein transport. Thus transport of a protein from the cytosol to the mitochondrial matrix requires: (i) a signal peptide attached to the NH_2 terminus of protein to be transported, (ii) a receptor protein at the outer membrane, (iii) ATP hydrolysis to supply energy and (iv) an electrochemical gradient.

For transport of a protein to mitochondrial matrix, the precursor protein has to first bind to a receptor protein that resides in the outer membrane. Later, it gets translocated to the matrix by crossing both outer and inner membranes, which join at certain contact sites to facilitate this process of simultaneous translocation across both the membranes. In a single mitochondrion, several such contact sites, where outer and inner membranes appear to be joined, have actually been observed under electron microscope and it is believed that translocation occurs near these contact sites. At these contact sites, there appear to be separate protein translocations in outer and inner membranes, whose functions are coupled to allow translocation across both the membranes at the same time. There is, however, evidence that the import process occurs in two stages. The first stage, involving insertion of signal peptide and adjoining sequences into both membranes, is not affected by low temperature (5°C) and is driven by the

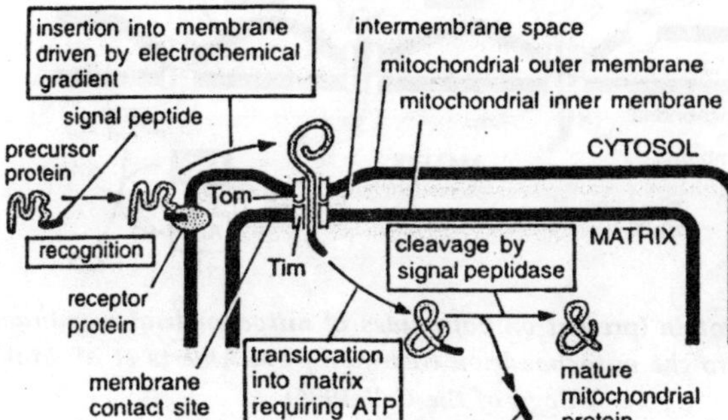

Protein import by mitochondria, utilizing signal peptide in the protein and a receptor in the mitochondrial membrane, (redrawn from Alberts et. al. Molecular, Biology of the Cell, 1994).

electrochemical gradient. The second stage involves movement of the remainder of the polypeptide chain into the matrix and requires ATP hydrolysis and a suitable temperature (25°C), so that at a low temperature, transport is arrested after the first stage (Fig.).

It has also been shown that cytosolic chaperone proteins (chaperonins) belonging to the hsp70 family also help in import of mitochondrial and ER proteins, by binding this protein in its unfolded state during translocation. These chaperonins also help in correct folding of cytosolic proteins. The hsp70 chaperonins are later released using ATP, thus accounting for dependence of later stages of import on ATP hydrolysis (Fig.). After an imported protein is released from hsp70, it is passed on to another chaperone protein, hsp60, which facilitates folding of protein inside the matrix. This sequential association of hsp70 and hsp60 also explains that proteins are imported into mitochondria in their unfolded state and get folded inside the matrix.

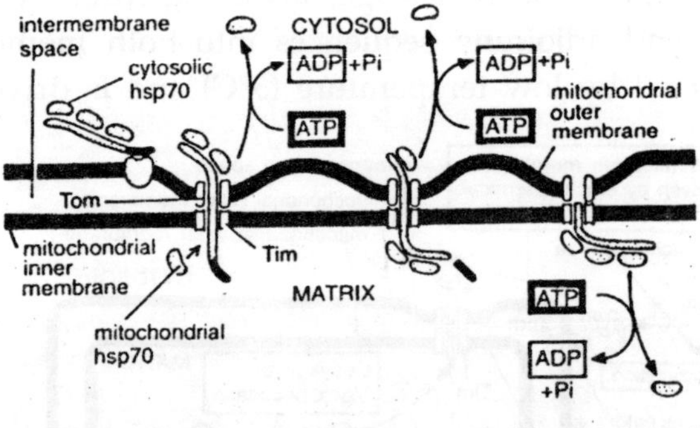

Role of hsp70 protein (present on both sides of mitochondrial membrane) in protein import into the mitochondrion (redrawn from Alberts et al. Molecular Bilogy of the Cell 1994)

Transport of Proteins into the Inner Membrane and Intermembrane Space of Mitochondria: The proteins targeted for the inner membrane or inter-membrane space are transported from the cytosol by the same mechanism, which is used for the transport of proteins to the matrix. These proteins may follow one of the two pathways: (i) they are prevented from completing the journey to the matrix and instead get localised in the intermembrane space/inner membrane; (ii) they may reach the matrix and are then transported back across the inner membrane to reach their final destination.

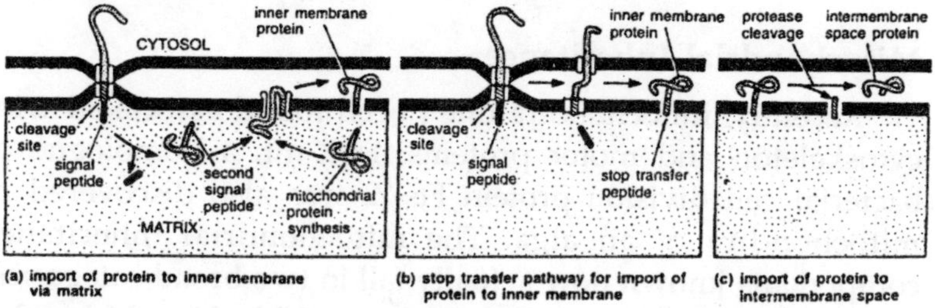

Pathways for the import of proteins from the cytosol into the intermembrane space of a mitochondrion (redrawn from Alberts et al. Molecular Biology of the Cell, 1994).

In the first direct pathway, a translocator in the inner membrane binds the hydrophobic sequence following the amino-terminal end of the signal peptide. The signal peptide is then cleaved off and' disintegrates in the matrix. The translocators in the outer and inner membrane become uncoupled, so that the protein is pulled into the intermembrane space and may remain attached to the inner membrane with the help of stop-transfer peptide. In case of proteins destined for the intermembrane space, the protein is cleaved off by a signal peptidase to release the mature soluble protein in the space. They may later become attached to the outer surface of the inner membrane (Fig.).

The Role

Mitochondria are often referred to as 'powerhouse' of the cell, since they produce 95% of ATP molecules in animal cells (5% ATP is produced during anaerobic respiration outside the mitochondria), although in plant cells, ATP is also produced by the chloroplasts. This energy is produced during the breakdown of food molecules including carbohydrates, fats and proteins (catabolic activity) which involves: (i) Embden-Meyerhof pathways (EMP or glycolysis); (ii) oxidative decarboxylation; and (iii) oxidative phosphorylation including: (a) Kreb's cycle or tricarboxylic acid (TCA) cycle; and (b) respiratory chain.

Mitochondrial Inheritance

Recently, mitochondira often been found associated with cytoskeleton and motor proteins. FtsZ-mt, a homologue of bacterial cell division protein Fts-Z, was also discovered in mitochondira of an alga. The mitochondrial inheritance components known now actually fall in two broad categories: (i) Cytosolic proteins (*e.g.* Mdmlp, Mdml4p, Mdm20p; FtsZ-mt), that remain associated with cytoskeleton and regulate mitochondrial distribution within a cell, (ii) Integral proteins of the mitochondrial outer membrane (*e.g.* Mdm10p, Mdml2p and Mdm l7), which may help in the attachment and interaction of mitochondria with cytoskeleton. The details of this machinery involved in the distribution and inheritance of mitochondria within a cell is beyond the scope of this book.

Evolutionary Origin of Mitochondrion

Monophyletic Origin of Mitochondrion from a Free Living Proteobacterium: Mitochondria resemble bacteria in many respects (Table) and are believed to have originated from some bacteria, rickettsial subdivision of the α-proteobacteria. During 1997-99, complete DNA sequences of bacteria like mitochondrial genome (*e.g. Reclinomonas americana;* 69,034 bp) and mitochondria like eubacterial genome (*e.g. Rickettsia prowazekii;* l,lll,523bp) have also been worked out, suggesting strongly that all extant mtDNAs had their origin in a single ancestral protomitochondrial genome, which in its turn, must have originated from a eubacterial genome (monophyletic origin rather than polyphyletic origin). A remarkable variation exists in the size of mtDNA and its gene content (Fig.). Based on this information, mtDNA has been classified in two basic types: (i) ancestral type with many genes as in *R. americana* and (ii) derived type marked with extensive gene loss, divergence in coding and non-coding DNA sequences, a new mitochondrial code, RNA editing, etc. (*e.g.* animal and fungal mtDNAs).

Comparison between Mammalian Mitochondria and Bacteria.

Characters	*Mitochondria*	*Bacteria*
1. Size: width length	0.2—1.0 μ 1.0—4 μ	0.2—2.0 μ 0.3—10.0 μ
2. Lipoprotein membrane	6—7 (nm)	7—8 (nm)
3. Invaginations of membrane	Cristae	Mesosomes
4. Respiratory control	Marked	Low or absent
5. Inhibitors of phosphorylion like CN—, CO, azide, antimycin, DNP and oligomycin	Effective	Less effective or ineffecive
6. DNA shape	Closed circle	Closed circle
7. Inhibitor of protein synthesis	Chloram-phenicol	Chloram-phenicol
8. Ribosomes	70S (variable)	70S

Simultaneous Origin of Eukaryotic Cells and Mitochondria ('Serial Endosymbiosis' vs 'Hydrogen Hypothesis'): A serial endosymbiosis model has also been proposed for the origin of nuclear genome and mitochondria. In this model, it is assumed that in the first step, the nuclear genome of the host itself resulted from the fusion of eubacterial and archaebacterial partners and that only in the second step, the mitochondrion was acquired as a symbiont. A group of eukaryotes known as

Archezoa, do lack mitochondria, suggesting that perhaps eukaryotes without mitochondria originated first as a primitive form and that the mitochondria entered the cells later.

The above view, however, has recently (1997-99) been challenged and it is suggested that the eukaryotes acquired the nucleus and mitochondria simultaneously, and that Archezoa (lacking mitochondria) must have resulted due to loss of mitochondria. This view was supported by the observation that genes for several mitochondrial proteins of bacterial origin are found in the genome of amitochondriate Archezoa and also in the organelle hydrogenosome, recently discovered in protists lacking mitochondria. This view is described as 'hydrogen hypothesis' since it assumes chimeric origin of eukaryotic nucleus, due to symbiotic association between a eubacterium (a proteobacterium, the symbiont), producing H_2 as the end product of anaerobic metabolism and a hydrogen-requiring autotrophic archaebacterium (the host). This hypothesis thus allows the possibility of simultaneous origin of the ancestor of eukaryotic cell and its mitochondrion (Fig.).

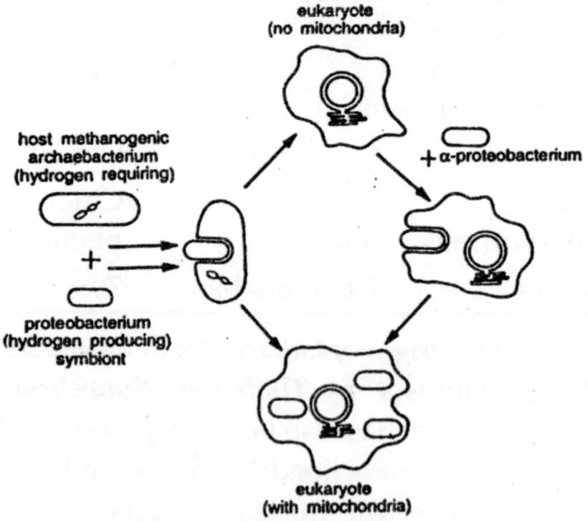

Two alternative hypotheses of the origin of eukaryotic cell and its mitochondrion.

7

Role of Protein

The total amount of DNA present in a cell may contain from a few to thousands of genes. Although the different types of cells in the body of a multicellular organism differ in structure and function, their genes are identical, since all the cells are ultimately derived from the zygote. The problem therefore is: how do cells with identical genetic complements differ so much in structure and function ? The answer is that not all genes are active at one time. As development proceeds certain genes become active while others become inactive, i.e. the genes are "switched on" and "switched off " at different times. This process is called *differential gene action.* When genes are active they direct the formation of enzymes which affect certain traits. The metabolic products formed may repress synthesis of enzymes *(feed-back or end product inhibition).* Thus enzyme synthesis is induced and repressed at different times.

Although a cell has the genes to produce hundreds of enzymes, only the enzymes required at a particular time are produced. This control mechanism ensures that the cell is not flooded with unnecessary enzymes. A hypothesis to explain induction and repression of enzyme synthesis was first put forward by Francois Jacob and Jacques Monod (1961) of the Institute Pasteur in Paris. For this and some other major contributions in biochemistry Jacob and Monod were awarded the Nobel Prize in Medicine in 1965. The scheme proposed by these workers is called the *operon model,* and has been considered to be the leading biological discovery of the present century, along with the elucidation of the structure of DNA by Watson and Crick (1953). The operon consists of the following components: *regulator gene, promoter gene* (a relatively recent concept), *operator gene, structural genes, repressor, corepressor* and *inducer.*

Constructional Genes

The structural genes direct synthesis of cellular proteins through messenger RNA (mRNA) and determine the sequence of amino acids in the proteins synthesised. There are as many structural genes in an operon as there are proteins or polypeptides under common control. Each structural gene may be controlled independently and transcribe a separate mRNA molecule, or all the structural genes of an operon may form one long *polycistronic* or *polygenic* mRNA molecule. Polygenic mRNAs are common in bacteria and bacteriophages. All known eukaryotes, however, contain only a single functional site for initiating protein synthesis.

The *lactose (lac) operon* of the bacterium *Escherichia coli* has been particularly well studied. It is a small segment of a circular DNA molecule which constitutes most of the genetic material of the bacterium. It has three structural genes, *z, y* and *a,* which transcribe one long polycistronic mRNA molecule. This controls the synthesis of three different proteins (enzymes), *β-galactosidase, galactoside permease* and *galactoside transacetylase.* These consist of 4, 1 and 2 units, respectively, *β-galactosidase* is the enzyme that splits lactose into glucose and galactose.

Galactoside permease facilitates the entry of lactose into the cell. *Galactoside acetylase* appears in small quantities upon lactose induction.

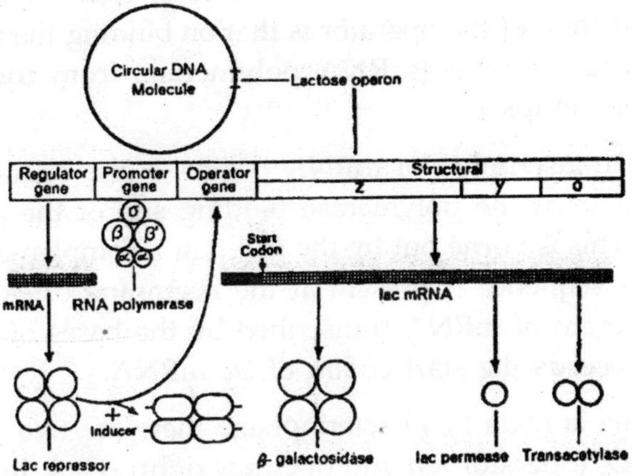

The lac operation of the bacterium Escherichia coli. Note the conformational change undergone by the lac repressor on addition of an inducer.

The *initiation codon* of structural gene z is TAC (corresponding to AUG of mRNA). It is located 10 base pairs away from the end of the operator gene.

In the bacterium *Salmonella typhimurium* the *histidine operon (histidon)* has 10 structural genes.

Manupulating Gene

The operator gene is adjacent to the first structural gene and controls the structural genes. It determines whether or not the structural genes are to be repressed by the *repressor*, a product of the regulator gene. The *operator* is recognised by the *repressor* protein which binds to the operator, forming an *operator-repressor* complex. Detailed studies of the bacterial *lac* operator and the two operators of the bacteriophage lambda (λ) have been carried out.

The *lac* operator of *E. coli* (Fig.) consists of a sequence of

35 nucleotide pairs. The base pairs in the operator show a two-fold symmetry *(palindromic sequences)*, which is also found in the promoter region. The operator gene binds one active *lac* repressor protein, which is a tetramer of four subunits. The basic function of the operator is that on binding the repressor it physically prevents RNA polymerase from forming in initiation complex.

The transcription of mRNA begins in the operator gene rather than at the polymerase binding site of the promoter region. This is borne out by the fact that a complementary *lac* operator sequence is present at the beginning of *lac* mRNA. The segment of mRNA transcribed by the bases of operator gene proceeds the start codon of *lac* mRNA.

In the lambda (λ) bacteriophage there are two *operators*, O_L and O_R (operator left and operator right) (Fig.). In contrast to the condition in the *lac* operator, the λ repressor binds to operators O_L and O_R at multiple successive sites (S_1 to S_6 and *S'_1 to S'_6)*. Of these the strongest binding sites, S_1 and S'_1, are the ones which are nearest to the first *structural* gene in the operon. One transcript starts with the *tof gene* which is adjacent to O_R and the other with the *N gene* which is adjacent to O_L. The repressor gene *cI* is located between O_L and O_R.

The same repressor protein recognises the two operators, O_L and O_R. The binding sites for the repressor on these two operators are, however, not identical. O_L and O_R have different base sequences. Several groups of base pairs in the S_1 site of O_L have a symmetrical arrangement, as in the *lac* repressor.

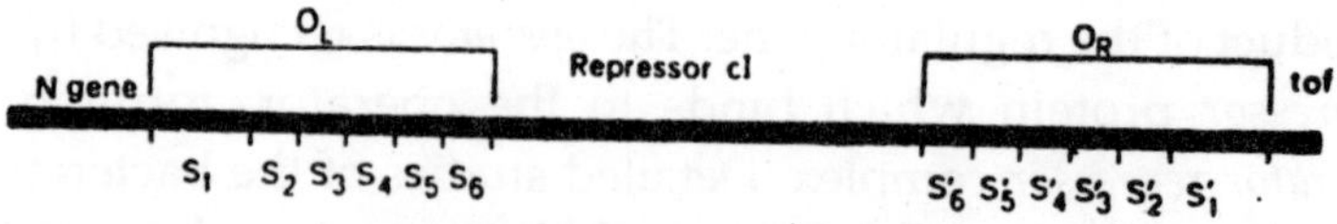

Operators of the lambda phage.

It has been seen that in the *lac* operator there is only a partial overlapping of the promoter and operator genes. In the lambda phage, however, the promoter site is located entirely within the operator. The promoter site includes the palindromic sequence: 5' G T C G A C 3' 3' C A G C T G 3'.

Elevative Gene

The promoter gene is continuous with the operator gene. The complete nucleotide sequence of the control region of the *lac* operon of *E. coli* has been worked out by Gilbert and Maxam (1973), Maziels (1973) and Dickson *et. al.* (1975) (Fig.). This sequence extends from the *termination codon* (ACT on DNA=UGA on mRNA) of the structural gene, and includes the promoter and operator genes.

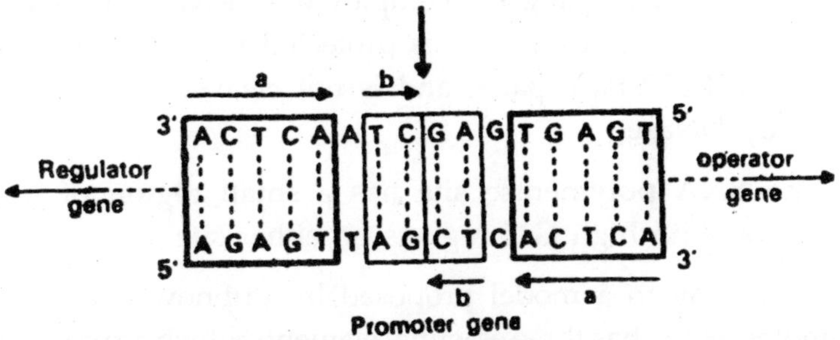

Part of the nucleotide sequence of the lac *promoter gene of* E. coli *showing the palindromic sequences a, b.*

The promoter region contains a *sequence of two-fold symmetry* in which sections of DNA on either site of a particular point (axis of twofold symmetry) are symmetrical. The sequences in these sections are *'palindromic'*. The nucleotides of one strand go in one direction, while an identical sequence of nucleotides goes in the opposite direction in the other strand. It has been suggested that these symmetrical regions of DNA may be recognised by proteins having symmetrically arranged subunits. The *CRP site* contains this section of two-fold symmetry. The CRP site binds a protein called CRP (*cyclic AMP receptor protein).* This protein is essential for the binding of the enzyme RNA polymerase to the promoter. The CRP is a dimer with two subunits and a molecular weight of 45,000. In *E. coli* the CRP combines with *cyclic adenesine monophosphate* (cAMP) to form a CRP-cAMP complex. This complex binds to the promoter. The CRP has a strong affinity for DNA, and this affinity increases considerably when the protein combines with cAMP. Binding of the CRP-cAMP complex to the promoter enhances RNA polymerase attachment to the promoter and thus increases transcription and protein synthesis. This is known as *positive control.*

It has been found that in *E.coli* and certain phages the RNA polymerase binds to DNA at the promoter site and forms a stable complex. If such DNA molecules are treated with pancreatic DNase (an enzyme which breaks down DNA), ihe region of DNA forming the complex with RNA is protected from the action of DNase. This protected region is found to consist of 40-50 base pairs, and is not cleaved into smaller pieces by DNase.

The RNA polymerase site has a small region of high A.T pairs, with high G.C regions on either site.

According to a model proposed by Pribnow (1975), the promoter region has three essential elements which are constant in position to each other (Fig.). These elements are: (i) a *recognition sequence* (ii) a *binding sequence* and (iii) an *mRNA initiation site.*

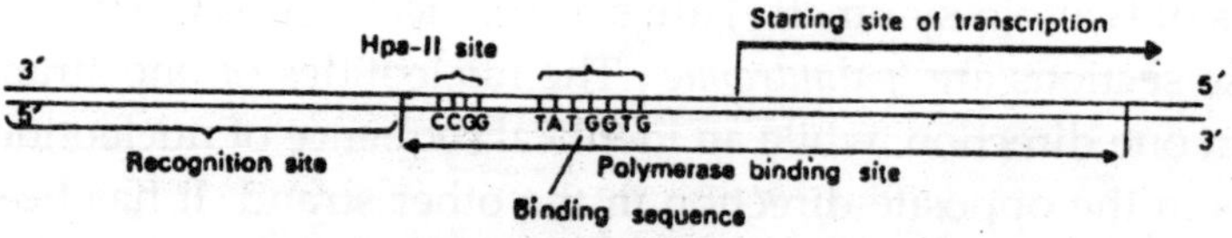

Diagram of E. coli promoter gene.

The *recognition sequence* is outside the polymerase binding site, i.e. the region of DNA protected against the action of DNase. According to the model, RNA polymerase first binds to DNA by forming a complex with the recognition sequence. It then binds with the binding sequence to produce the *pre-initiation complex.*

The *binding site* consists of a sequence of seven bases. These are present in a constant location in the protected fragments. The sequence of this set of seven bases has been found to be almost constant in the bacteria and phages studied. It never differs by more than two bases from the following sequence: 5' TATPuATG.

RNA initiation site. The start of mRNA transcription takes place on one of two bases near the binding sequence. This starting site is included in the DNA fragment protected from DNase digestion. In the *lac* operon there is overlapping of promoter and operator sites. At least a part of the operator sequences appear in the polymerase binding site sequences.

In the promoter region, 20 base pairs to the left of the starting site of transcription, is a sequence 5′CCGG. This is the substrate for an endonuclease enzyme isolated from *Hemophilus parainfluenzae,* and is know as the Hpa II site. This site has been used as a reference point in studies of repressor and polymerase binding.

Organisms		*RNA polymerase binding sequence ('Constant' 7 bases)*		*Start of transcription mRNA* →	
fd	5′......A C	U A U A A U A	G A C A G	G G	U A A A..3′
T7A3	.....G G	U A C G A U G	U A C C A	C A	U G A A...
T7A2	....A G	U A A G A U A	C A A A U	C G	C U A A...
UV-5	.....C G	U A U A A U G	U G U G G	A A	U U G U...
λP_R	....G U	G A U A A U G	G U U G C	A U	G U A C...

Sequences of RNA transcripts of different micro-organisms coded by double-stranded DNA. Bases in boldface indicate start of transcription. The RNA polymerase binding sequence consists of 'constant' 7 bases. These constant bases are transcribed by a DNA sequence which never differs by more than two bases from 5′ TATPuATG.

Regulator Gene

The regulator gene directs the synthesis of a protein, which may be an *active repressor* or an *inactive repressor (aporepressor)*. In the *inducible system* the active repressor formed has an affinity for the operator gene. In the absence of an inducer (Figs.) the *lac* repressor protein binds to the operator gene and blocks the path of RNA polymerase. Thus the structural genes are unable to transcribe mRNA, and protein synthesis does not take place. In the presence of an *inducer,* (e.g. *lactose)* the repressor protein binds to the inducer to form an *inducer-repressor-complex* (Fig.B). Each repressor subunit has one binding site for the inducer. The repressor undergoes a conformational change which makes it inactive. It cannot now bind to the operator gene, and hence the structural genes can synthesise proteins.

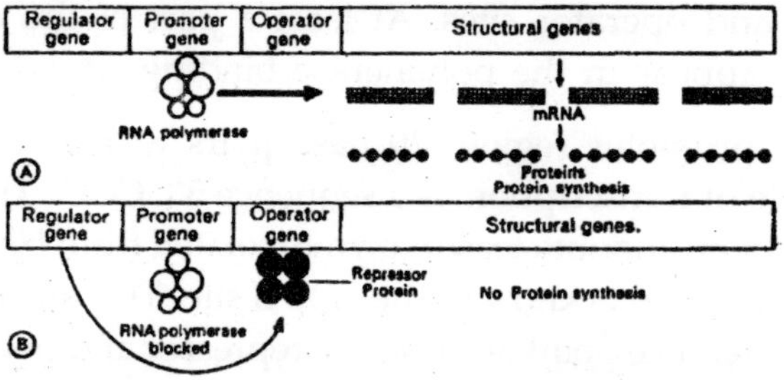

The promoter gene. (A) Binding of RNA polymerase to promoter gene. RNA polymerase moves along the structural genes catalysing synthesis of proteins. (B) Repressor protein formed by the regulator gene binds to the operator gene. Movement of RNA polymerase is blocked, and hence no protein synthesis takes place.

In the *repressible system* the repressor protein formed by the regulator gene is inactive and does not block the operator (Fig.). The structural genes, therefore synthesise proteins. The repressor is activated in the presence of a *corepressor,* and the *repressor-corepressor* complex blocks the operator gene (Fig.). The structural genes, therefore, cannot synthesise proteins.

In the *lac* operon of *E.coli* the repressor protein produced by the regulator gene consists of four subunits, each of 40,000 daltons, and has 347 amino acid residues. The active repressor protein has a strong affinity for a segment of the operator gene composed of 12-15 nucleotides.

Types of Control Mechanisms: The control of protein

synthesis by regulator proteins may be by *induction* or *repression*. There may also be *negative* or *positive control.*

Induction: A category of enzymes called *inducible enzymes* are normally absent from the cell or are present in very small quantities. They increase in quantity only in the presence of an *inducer*. Such a system is called an *inducible system.* A bacterial culture of *E.coli* growing in a medium with glucose as the source of carbon produces only minute quantities of the enzyme β-*galactosidase.* Only one or two molecules of the enzyme are present. When *lactose* is added to the medium the production of β-galactosidase starts, and within two to three minutes about 3,000 molecules are synthesised by the Z gene. β-*galactosidase* hydrolyses lactose into the sugars galactose and glucose. Some galactose and glucose molecules are converted into *allolactose,* which is the inducer for β-galactosidase synthesis.

In the *lac* system *allolactose* is the *actual inducer* while *lactose* is the *apparent inducer.* An artificial inducer commonly used an experimental work is *isopropylthiogalactoside* (IPTG).

When the *inducer is absent* the active *repressor* protein produced by the *regulator gene* associates with the *operator gene* and blocks it. No transcription of mRNA by the structural genes can therefore take place, and hence there is no enzyme synthesis. Absence of the inducer may be due to the fact that is not present in the growth medium or is not synthesised by the micro-organism.

When the *inducer is present* the active repressor binds to the inducer molecule to form a *repressor-inducer complex* (R-I). A conformational change takes place in the repressor molecule which is inactivated. This prevents binding to the operator, which is therefore not blocked. The structural genes transcribe mRNA, and enzyme synthesis takes place.

Repression: The synthesis of an enzyme may be inhibited by a product of metabolism. In *E. coli* tryptophan synthetase is inhibited by tryptophan. Thus tryptophan synthetase is formed only if the bacterium is grown in a tryptophan free medium. The amino acid *histidine* also acts as a repressor. This process is called *enzyme repression.* In the repressible system the protein produced by the regulator gene is an *inactive repressor,* also called the *aporepressor.* The aporepressor on combining with a *corepressor* or *effector* molecule becomes activated. It undergoes a conformational change which enables it to bind to the operator gene.

When the *corepressor is absent* the inactive aporepressor does not bind to the operator gene. Because the operator gene is not blocked, the structural genes transcribe mRNA, and protein synthesis takes place.

When the *corepressor is present* the aporepressor combines with it to form a complex, and is activated. The complex blocks the operator gene. The structural genes are therefore unable to synthesise mRNA, and consequently no protein synthesis takes place. The corepressor may be a product of one of the enzymes produced by the structural genes.

Regulation of Enzyme Synthesis by Induction and Repression.

Inducible System

1. ***Inducer absent:*** Regulator gene → Active repressor.

   → Binds to and blocks operator gene.

   → No mRNA transcription by structural genes.

   → No enzyme synthesis.

2. ***Inducer present:*** Regulator gene → Active repressor

   → + inducer → Inactive repressor.

   → No blocking of operator gene.

   → mRNA transcription by structural genes.

   → Enzyme synthesis.

Repressive System

1. ***Corepressor Absent:*** Regulator gene → Inactive repressor (aporepressor)

   → No blocking of operator gene.

   → mRNA transcription by structural genes.

   → Enzyme synthesis.

2. ***Corepressor Present:*** Regulator gene → Inactive repressor (aporepressor)

   → + corepressor → Active repressor.

   → Binds to and blocks operator gene.

   → No mRNA transcription by structural genes.

   → No enzyme synthesis.

Negative Control: It has been seen that both in the inducible and repressible systems, protein synthesis takes place when the operator gene is free and stops when it is blocked. Gene expression therefore only takes place when the operator gene is free. Such a control mechanism for protein synthesis is thus of the *negative type.* An example of negative control is the induction of protein synthesis in the presence of lactose and absence of glucose by the *lac* operon of *E. coli.*

In negative control the regulator protein is the *repressor* and it *prevents gene transcription.* The controlling site on the operon is the *operator gene.* In the *inducible system* the effector molecule is the *inducer.* The inducer prevents repressor function and thus enables gene transcription and protein synthesis. In the *repressible system* the effector molecule is the *corepressor.* The corepressor stimulates repression function and thus prevents gene transcription.

Positive Control: In positive control the regulator protein acts as an *activator* and increases enzyme synthesis. The activator attaches to a separate controlling site, the *initiator site,* on DNA.

The initiator site is not necessarily the operator gene. Since the regulator protein enhances gene transcription, this type of regulation is called *positive control* of protein synthesis.

The *ara* operon of *E. coli* (Fig.), which functions in the utilisation of *arabinose,* is an example of positive control. The first three genes of the *ara* operon are *ara* D, *ara* A and *ara* B. These genes specify the synthesis of an *epimerase,* an *isomerase* and a *kinase,* respectively. An associated gene, *ara* C, functions as a *regulator gene.* The *ara* C gene may act as both *activator* and *repressor.* The *regulator protein* produced by the *ara* C gene may combine with *arabinose (inducer)* to form an *activator* protein. This activator protein binds to the *initiator site (ara* I) on the operon and enhances enzyme synthesis. In the absence of arabinose the regulator protein of *ara* C binds to the *operator* site (*ara* O), and thus acts as a *repressor.*

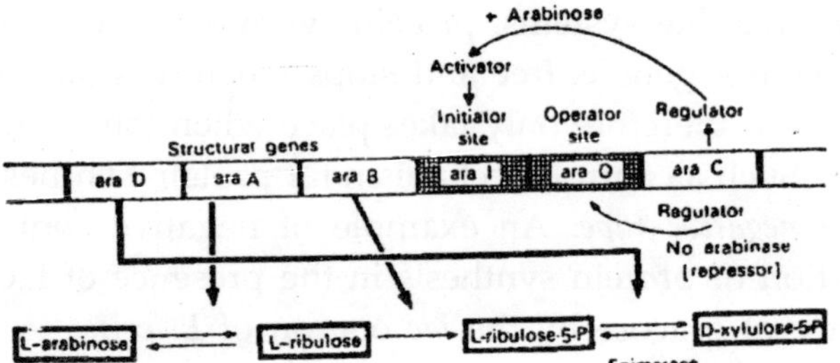

The L-arabinose operon of E. coli.

Replication of DNA is an important example of positive control. Bacterial chromosomes consist of replicating units called *replicons* which are capable of independent genetic replication. One of the structural genes of the replicon produces an *activator* which is influenced by cytoplasmic stimuli. The activator interacts with the *replicator,* a particular section of the replicon, and initiates replication at this point.

Positive control may also be of the *inducible* or *repressible* type. In the *inducible system,* the effector molecule is the *inducer.* The inducer stimulates activator function and enables gene transcription and protein synthesis. In the *repressible system* the effector molecule is the *corepressor*. The corepressor prevents activator function, and thus gene transcription.

Succession in the Operon

Regulator Gene: A mutation taking place in a regulator gene may produce a non-functional repressor protein with a changed amino acid sequence. Such mutants are called *constitutive mutants*. A mutant repressor is not able to bind to the operator gene. Under such conditions the action of RNA polymerase would not be blocked. The structural genes transcribe mRNA and enzyme synthesis occurs regardless of need. Such enzymes are called *constitutive enzymes*.

Promoter Gene: A mutation in the promoter may either totally prevent attachment of RNA polymerase, or may increase or decrease attachment. When attachment is totally prevented, the structural genes cannot transcribe mRNA and there is no enzyme synthesis. An "up-promoter" mutation which permits more rapid attachment of RNA polymerase molecules results in an increased rate of enzyme synthesis. Conversely, a "down-promoter" mutation which decreases the rate of RNA polymerase attachment results in reduced enzyme synthesis. There are also some promoter mutations which reduce the requirement of cyclic AMP.

Regulation of Gene Activity in Eukaryotes: Genes are active only when their products are required by the cell. The rest of the time they are 'switched off'. Thus in mouse liver cells only about 3% of the genes are active (i.e. transcribe RNA), and in brain cells about 9% are turned on.

In prokaryotes control of gene activity takes place by means of special *repressor proteins* transcribed by *regulator genes*. Binding of the repressor protein to the *operator gene* blocks the movement of the transcribing enzyme *RNA polymerase*, and thus prevents RNA transcription by the *structural genes*.

In eukaryotes gene regulation takes place by a different mechanism. The possible candidates for regulation of gene activity are the proteins associated with DNA in the chromosomes. These include *histones* and *non-histone chromosomal proteins* (NHC proteins). It is unlikely that histones *selectively* repress gene activity since they have almost identical amino acid compositions in different organisms. It has been suggested that histones probably mask DNA in a *nonspecific* manner *(non-specific repression).*

Because histones are rich in *lysine* and *arginine* they have a *net positive charge* and are basic proteins. The positively charged groups, which appear to be arranged in clusters, could interact with the *negative charge* of the *phosphate backbone of DNA*. This would greatly reduce the charge repulsion of the phosphate groups and would facilitate *supercoiling of DNA*. The *RNA polymerase* molecule would not be able to move along the supercoiled DNA, and thus no transcription would be possible. It is thus possible that histones prevent transcription by bringing about supercoiling of DNA. This is shown by the fact that incorporation of RNA precursors in eukaryote cells take place only in regions of the chromosome where the chromatin is diffuse and not in the highly compact regions. The highly compact heterochromatic regions of the chromosome are therefore inert and cannot carry out transcription.

Among the models proposed to explain gene regulation in higher cells are: (i) Frenster's (1965) model of gene-specific *derepressor RNA,* (ii) models in which *non-histone proteins* act as derepressors, e.g. those proposed by Paul and co-workers (1971) and Stein *et at* (1975) and (iii) Britten and Davidson's *operon-aperator model* (1969).

Frenster's Model: Histones stabilize the DNA double helix by interacting with the negative phosphate groups of DNA. This prevents the separation of strands, and consequently transcription. The histones thus act as general *repressors* of protein synthesis. Histones are displaced from DNA by nuclear polyions which form complexes with histones. This permits separation of the DNA strands in a random manner. Gene-specific *derepressor RNA* hybridises with the non-transcribing DNA strand at a particular locus and stabilises the loop in the open position. This frees the other DNA strand and permits it to transcribe messenger RNA.

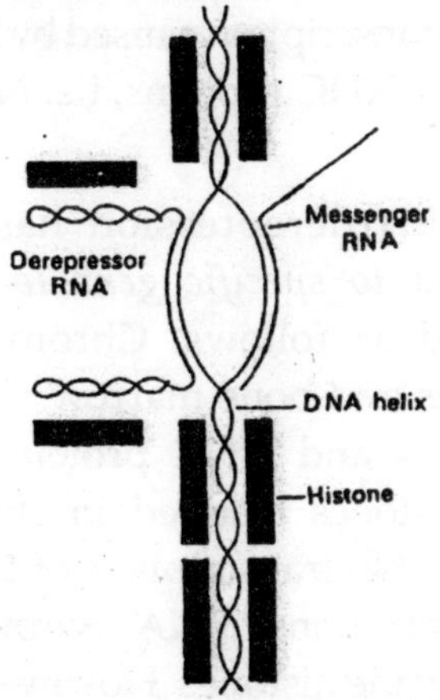

Frenster's model of gene regulation.

Nonhistone Proteins as Derepressors: Paul and co-workers (1971) have suggested a similar model, except that in their model gene-specific *acid proteins* displace the histone. The *nonhistone chromosomal proteins* have a number of characteristics expected of a regulatory protein with specific action.

(1) NHC proteins occur in a far greater variety of forms than histones. They differ greatly in size and the length of the time they are associated with DNA before degradation.

(2) The pattern of NHC proteins varies from species to species. Even different tissues in the same organism differ in their NHC protein pattern.

(3) The pattern of NHC proteins varies with the developmental stage and also with the stage of the cell

cycle. Thus NHC proteins isolated from interphase cells, where transcription of RNA is maximal, differ from those isolated from metaphasic cells, where only a few genes transcribe RNA.

(4) NHC proteins have been localised in the active regions of the chromosomes.

(5) Inhibition of transcription caused by histones is reversed on addition of NHC proteins, i.e. NHC proteins act as *derepressors.*

(6) Moreover, this derepression has *specificity.* NHC proteins *bind to specific gene loci.* This has been demonstrated as follows. Chromatin isolated from rabbit thymus and bone marrow was dissociated into DNA, histones and NHC protein. Re-association of DNA and histones resulted in chromatin free from NHC protein. No transcription of RNA was observed in such preparations. RNA synthesis is completely suppressed by the histones. However, addition of NHC proteins from bone marrow resulted in transcription of RNA with characteristics of that of bone marrow. Similarly, addition of thymus NHC proteins resulted in RNA with characteristics of that found in thymus cells. This shows that NHC proteins are specific for a cell type. It is presumed that NHC proteins derepress specific genes and stimulate transcription of specific genetic regions.

In another test this specificity is even more clearly demonstrated. Foetal mouse liver cells synthesise the protein *globin* (the non-iron part *of haemoglobin)* but foetal mouse brain cells do not. *In vitro* addition of NHC proteins from foetal liver to DNA and histone from the brain leads to production of globin mRNA.

(7) NHC proteins show preferential binding to the DNA of the organisms from which they are isolated.

According to the theory of Stein and his co-workers (see Stein, G.S., Stein J.S. and Klein smith, 1975), regulation of gene activity takes place as follows (Fig.). Histones probably act as *nonspecific repressors* of genetic function and prevent transcription of RNA from DNA. Individual NHC proteins recognise certain sites on DNA and bind to it there. They then pull off the histone repressor from the site, thus *derepressing DNA*. NHC proteins act by de-repressing.

The Britten-Davidson (1969) operon-operator model (Fig.) for regulation in higher cells includes certain features which are not found in the simpler Jacob-Monod model for bacterial cells. According to this speculative model four basic types of genes are visualised, *sensor genes, producer genes, integrator genes* and *receptor genes.*

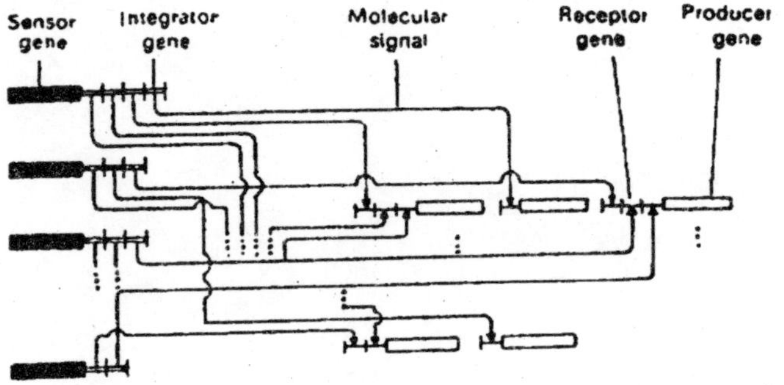

The Britten-Davidson generalised 'operon-operator' model for gene regulation in eukaryotic cells.

1. Sensor genes are detectors which are sensitive to the state of the cell and its environment. The sensor gene is stimulated by various substances like enzymes, hormones and metabolities, perhaps through intermediary molecules.
2. Producer genes are the output controls of the regulation mechanism. They specify controls for the formation of cell structures like membranes, organells, etc., and operator substances like enzymes, etc.

3. An integrator gene may be associated with a sensor gene, or several integrators may be associated with a sensor. The integrator gene sends out a specific signal (molecule) to other genes when the sensor gene is activated. When several integrators are associated with a single sensor, the sensor can initiate a variety of signals.
4. A receptor gene is associated with a single producer gene, and is a link between the integrator gene and the producer gene. When the receptor gene receives an integrator signal the producer gene is activated. A particular producer gene may have many receptors associated with it.

8

Locating Genes

In 1928 Belling suggested that the chromomeres, which appear like a series of granules on the chromosome, might be the genes. Although the view received little support at that time, some recent work tends to support the view that the chromomeres represent the sites of genes. Whole mounts of meiotic chromosomes show chromomeres under the electron microscope.

The chromosomes consist of *axial filaments* from which arise *chromatin fibre loops*. In the region of the chromomeres there is increased density in the attachment of the loops to the axial filaments. Callan and Llyod (1960) have suggested that each loop of lampbrush chromosomes is correlated with the activity of a gene.

According to them the loop may possibly contain several identical *'slave genes'* controlled by a *'master gene'* (Fig.). Thomas (1969) has also suggested that each chromomere represents a functional gene, i.e. a master gene with many slave copies.

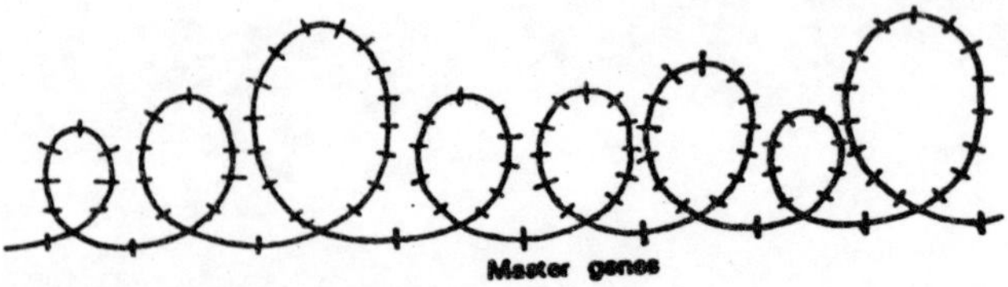

Diagram showing the master gene' and 'slave gene' concept of Callan and Lloyd.

Beerman's (1967) work on mutations supports the view that in polytene chromosomes the dark bands (which represent transverse rows of chromomeres) correspond to genes. It has, however, been pointed out by Watson (1970) that the interband region of polytene chromosomes must also contain genes.

There is, however, no one-to-one correspondence between chromomeres and genes. For example, it has been estimated that the total number of chromomeres in one set of chromosomes of man is at the most 600. The total number of known mutations in man is, however, much greater than this (McKusik, 1971). Thus the view that each chromomere represents a functional gene is not tenable. Coming (1972) has suggested that chromomeres may represent families of related genes, or at least genes having similar base compositions.

The first picture of an isolated gene was published by Shapiro and co-workers in 1969. They chemically purified the *lac* operon of DNA and photographed it with the help of an electron microscope.

In Almost all Cases Genes are DNA. The genes of almost all organisms are DNA. This is shown by the following observations.

(1) Genetic *transformation* experiments of Avery, Macleod and McCarty (1944) first clearly established the role of DNA as genetic material, and gave evidence of the chemical nature of the gene. DNA was isolated from a virulent strain of bacteria. An avirulent strain was

grown in a medium containing this DNA. After some time virulent bacteria could be isolated from the medium. These could reproduce indefinitely, producing virulent strains.

It is apparent that genes (DNA) from the virulent strain when introduced into the avirulent strain transformed the latter into the virulent strain. When DNase, an enzyme which breaks down DNA, was added to the medium no transformation occurred. This confirmed the fact that transformation was due to DNA and not because of any impurities.

(2) Chromosomes contain DNA, proteins (mostly histones) and varying amounts of RNA. It is unlikely that genes are made of proteins since the proteins associated with sperm heads differ in composition from histones of other tissues. Similarly, RNA cannot be the genetic material since sperms contain negligible amounts of RNA. It therefore follows that DNA must be the genetic material.

(3) The DNA content of all cells of a species of an organism is constant. It is halved in the gametes.

(4) Cells of similar hereditary origin have DNA of similar composition. The relative amounts of the four nucleotides are constant.

(5) Gene mutations can be explained on the basis of alteration of DNA structure.

The Genes of some Viruses are RNA: Most plant viruses and some animal viruses contain RNA as the genetic material. In the Reo group of viruses and in the wound tumour virus the RNA is present in the double stranded from. In the tobacco mosaic virus (TMV), A tobacco virus, influenza Type A virus, and bacterial viruses F2, R17 and MS2 the RNA is single-stranded.

The Genome and the Plasmon: The total hereditary material may be divided into the *genome* and the *plasmon*. The *genome* is the hereditary material of the chromosomal complex. The *plasmon* is the total hereditary material outside the chromosome. The term plasmon was introduced by Fritz von Wettstein in 1924. The smallest heritable unit of the plasmon is the *plasmagene*, a term introduced by Darlington in 1939. Plasmagenes are known by different names according to their location in different cell structures. The plasmagenes of plastids are called *plastogenes*, those of kinetosomes *kinetogenes*, those of mitochondria *chondriogenes* and those of centrioles *centriogenes*.

The gene has been variously considered as a unit of recombination *(recon)*, a unit of mutation *(muton)* and a unit of function *(cistron)*. These three units are not identical.

The Gene as a Unit of Recombination (recon): On the basis of work on *Drosophila* the gene was considered to be the shortest segment of a chromosome which could be separated from its adjacent segments during crossing over. It was thought that genes were those parts of the chromosomes *between* which crossing over could take place. Crossing over was, however, not supposed to take place *within* the genes. The gene was thought to be an *indivisible unit* of a chromosome controlling some phenotypic character. However, on the basis of tests for recombinations it has been shown that in viral DNA strands, crossing over not only takes place between the genes but also within genes. One of the subunits of the gene has been called the *recon*. It is the smallest unit capable of recombining genetically. Recombination studies on microbes indicate that structurally the recon consists of one or two pairs of nucleotides, possibly only one pair.

That crossing over takes place within the gene was demonstrated by Benzer (1955, etc.) in the T4 bacteriophage. Before this it was thought that crossing over could take place only between genes. When bacteriophage cultures are grown on agar plates they form colonies or *plaques* on the plate (Fig.). *Normal* wild type bacteriophages form plaques with smooth edges. *Mutant* bacteriophages, called rII, form larger, rough-edged plaques. Benzer found that two adjacent genes, rIIA and rIIB were responsible for the rough-edged plaque trait.

Each gene forms a polypeptide, and the two polypeptides form the protein. A change (mutation) in either polypeptide chain would result in phenotypic expression. Genetic mapping has shown that in the rIIA gene there are at least 500 mutational sites where crossing- over is possible (Fig.). If crossing over occurs within the gene, then by mating two rII mutants it should be possible to form the normal wild type. Benzer found that this was indeed the case. He calculated that the lowest frequency of cross-over was 0.02% and found that crossing-over occurs between two adjacent nucleotides of DNA. Thus, the unit of recombination (recon) is much smaller than the unit of function (cistron).

The Gene as a Unit of Mutation (Muton): The gene has also been defined from the point of view of mutation. The shortest chromosomal unit capable of undergoing mutation has been called the *muton*. The muton consists of one or many pairs of nucleotides within the DNA molecule. In many cases a gene mutation is a change in a single nucleotide unit of DNA.

The Gene as Unit of Function (Cistron): In 1908 Garrod first proposed the *one-gene-one-enzyme* hypothesis. This concept was clearly demonstrated by Beadle and Tatum in 1941. The gene was considered to be the unit for coding the synthesis of a single enzyme. It was thus identified by its functional product, the enzyme. The one-gene-one-enzyme hypothesis has been expressed in several different ways. Since the gene forms a messenger RNA molecule it can also be said that *one gene forms one messenger RNA*. In some cases, however, several genes form a single mRNA strand, which is then said to be *polycistronic.* The concept has also been expressed as *one-gene-one-protein,* since the messenger RNA molecule serves for coding of a protein (enzyme). It would be more correct to use the statement *one-gene-one-polypeptide chain,* since an enzyme or protein may contain more than one polypeptide chain. The chains formed by different genes then aggregate to form the enzyme (protein molecule). Stahl has defined the gene as a *polynucleotide chain consisting of segments, each controlling the expression of a particular trait.*

The functional gene has been called the cistron by Benzer because it is a chromosomal segment within which the cis-trans effect operates. The cistron represents a segment of the DNA molecule, and consists of a linear sequence of nucleotides which controls some cellular functions. In most cases the cistron is approximately equivalent to the gene of the geneticist. In *E. coli* the cistron may contain about 1,500 base pairs. There is evidence that some cistrons may contain as many as 30,000 nucleotide pairs. Because the genetic code is a triplet one, a protein consisting of *n* amino acids is coded by a cistron of about 3*n* nucleotides. The cistron starts with an *initiating codon* and ends with a *terminating codon.* Each cistron is responsible for coding one messenger RNA molecule, which in turn serves for the formation of a polypeptide chain. It has been found that hundreds of units of mutation (mutons) and recombination (recons) exist within each cistron. Cistrons, therefore, occupy a much greater chromosomal length than mutons or recons.

The T4 virus (bacteriophage) contains a single long DNA molecule lying within a protein head. The DNA molecule has several regions, one of which is called the rII region (Fig.). Benzer (1955, 1956) has studied the rII region and has found that it consists of two cistrons, A and B. Each of these regions can function independently and contains 2,500 and 1,500 nucleotide pairs respectively. Each cistron contains several small units of mutation and recombination.

Number of Genes

The number of genes that an organism possesses has some relationship to its complexity. Viruses are parasitic on host cells. They produce messenger RNA but depend on the host cell for transfer RNA, ribosomal RNA and some enzymes. Consequently they require very few genes. The bacteriophages R17 and Q *B* have RNA as their genetic material. The single-stranded RNA contains only three genes. One codes for *A protein,* the second for *coat protein,* and the third for one of four subunits of *replicase.* (The other three units of replicase are host proteins).

Polyoma or SV40 viruses have 5-10 genes and their chromosomes are only 1.7 microns in length. The single-stranded DNA virus ϕX174 has DNA which codes for 9 proteins. The bacterial virus lambda (λ) has about 40 genes and T4 has over a hundred genes. The number of genes in viruses ranges from only three in the simplest viruses to about 250 in the most complex ones.

Although there is some relationship between the number of genes and the complexity of an organism, there in no strict correlation between apparent genetic complexity and the DNA content per haploid nucleus. Thus, some fishes and amphibians contain 10 to 20 times more DNA than humans. Moreover, the size of the genome varies over a 20-fold range within the species of a phylum.

In *Escherichia coli* the chromosome is about 1 mm long and contains about 4,000 genes, and 4,000,000 base pairs. The total number of genes in *Drosophila melanogaster* is estimated to be 5,000 on the basis of observation of bands in salivary gland chromosomes.

The normal diploid human cell contains about 5 picograms (5×10^{-12}) of DNA. This is equivalent to 5×10^{9} (5 billion) base pairs. Assuming that the average gene contains 1,000 base pairs, the number of genes in the haploid human cell would be 5×10^6 (5 million). This number is probably too high, at least by a factor of 10, because all DNA is not used for coding proteins.

Number of Nucleotides in the Average Gene: It is possible to find out the number of nucleotides in a gene if the molecular weight of the gene is known, since each base pair has a molecular weight of about 600. Thus in the bacteriophage T4, which has over a 100 genes and a chromosomal molecular weight of 120 million, each gene has an average MW of 1.2 million. Now, since the molecular weight of a pair of bases is about 600 the average gene should contain about 2,000 base pairs. However, all the genes of T4 are not known. Assuming that the total number of genes will at maximum be doubled, the average gene would have 900-1500 base pairs.

The F2 RNA virus contains-only 3,000 nucleotides which can code for about 1,000 amino acids. The tobacco necrosis virus contains still fewer nucleotides, about 1000, which are just sufficient to code for the average-sized protein molecule. The necrosis virus invades a host cell along with another RNA virus (with about 6,000 nucleotide), and uses the enzymes of the larger virus for its replication.

Duplication of Genes: Genes are segments of the DNA molecule. It therefore follows that the genes will undergo duplication when the DNA molecule replicates. This takes place during the interphase preceeding mitosis. The two strands of the DNA double helix separate from each other. To each strand are attached nucleotides that were present in the former partner *(complementary pairing)*. In this way two identical double strands of DNA are formed. In sexually-reproducing forms all the cells in the body have been ultimately derived from the zygote, and therefore normally have identical gene sets.

Gene Action: Genes act by controlling the structure and rate of production of specific proteins (enzymes). The DNA of each gene forms a complementary mRNA strand, which attaches to the ribosomes. Here it serves for arranging tRNA molecules in a specific sequence. Each tRNA molecule brings with it a specific amino acid.

Thus the sequence of amino acids (i.e. the structure of the protein or enzyme) is determined by the sequence of nucleotides in mRNA. This in turn is determined by the sequence of nucleotides in DNA (gene). A series of enzyme-controlled reactions determine traits in an organism. Since the structure of these enzymes is controlled by the genes it follows that genes determine traits. The whole chain of events may be summarised as follows:

DNA → mRNA → Sequence of amino acids → Traits.
(gene) (structure of enzymes)

Gene Regulation: Jacob and Monod (1961) proposed the *operon model* to explain the control of gene activity. It was assumed that there are three kinds of genes, *structural genes, operator genes* and *regulator genes. Structural genes* are those that produce mRNA. *Operator genes* control structural genes by acting as switches in controlling mRNA synthesis by the latter. These different types of genes together constitute the *operon. Regulator genes* produce substances *(repressers)* which block the operator genes, so that mRNA synthesis by structural genes is prevented.

Loci and Alleles: A gene occupies a definite position within the chromosome. This position is called the *locus*. Since chromosomes exist in homologous pairs, each cell contains two kinds of genes which are found in pairs. The two members of a pair of genes are called *alleles* (the old term was *allellomorphs).* Usually alleles are alike, but sometimes they may differ. A fertilized egg may have a gene for brown eyes from one parent and a gene for black eyes from another. The genes for a particular trait need not necessarily be together. In *Drosophila* the genes for eye colour are scattered about among all the chromosomes.

Separate Genes

It was formerly believed that a gene coding the synthesis of a particular polypeptide had a continuous sequence of nucleotides. Among the first reports indicating that the DNA sequence coding for a polypeptide is not present continuously were provided by the *'hexon' gene* of adenovirus and the *ovalbumin gene* of chickens.

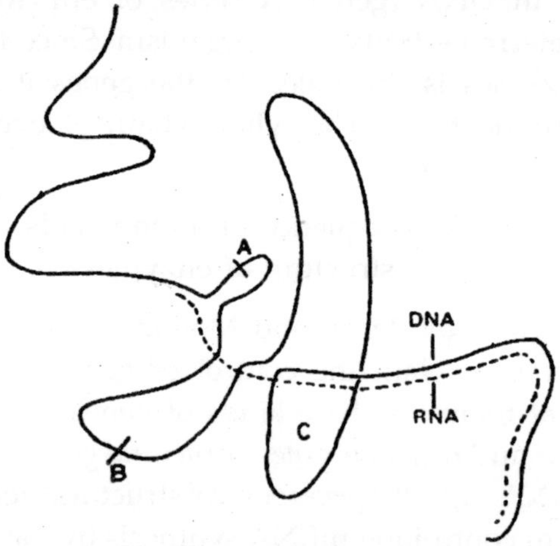

The hexon gene of adenovirus with its transcribed mRNA. The loops (A, B, C) represent regions of DNA which do not transcribe RNA.

Hexon Gene (Fig.): The DNA of adenovirus is double-stranded and codes for about 20 proteins. Eight of the genes are called 'late genes' because they transcribe mRNA late in the virus' life. The eight late genes transcribe a single RNA which is later cut into eight mRNAs. The total length of the eight mRNAs is, however, less than the length of the original transcript. When one (the hexon gene) of the eight genes was paired with its mRNA the DNA formed three *loops* which represent the *unpaired regions.* This indicated that the hexon mRNA was transcribed by four different regions (unlooped regions), and that the four segments were then joined together. The looping is obviously a device to exclude unwanted DNA which does not transcribe RNA.

Ovalbumin Gene (Fig.): P. Chambon's group (France) and B. W. O'Malley's group (USA) showed that the *ovalbumin gene* of chickens is not contiguous but is made up of pieces scattered in the chromosome. Such genes have been called *split genes.* Within a gene there may be silent regions which are not represented in the polypeptide chain. The natural ovalbumin gene transcribes precursor RNA which contains intervening sequences not found in mRNA. The precursor RNA loops out these intervening sequences, which are then excised, to form mRNA.

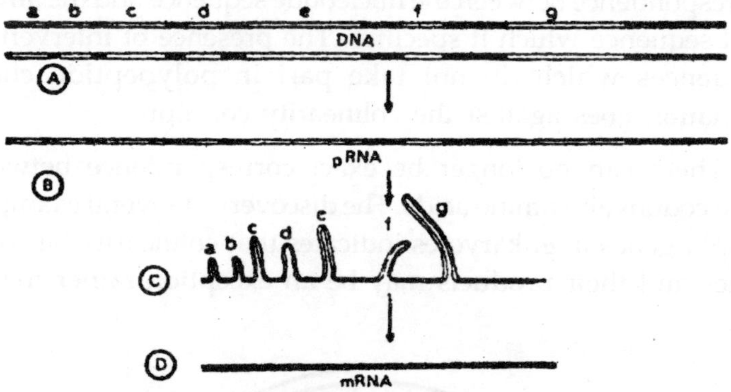

Transcription and processing of mRNA of the ovalbumin gene.

A. ***Ovalbumin gene with coding sequences (black) and noncoding sequences (white, a-g).***

B. ***Precursor RNA (pRNA) transcribed by DNA.***

C. ***Non-coding sequences of pRNA loop out.***

D. ***mRNA after excision of loops. Reports of split genes have been obtained from other sources, e.g. β-globin genes of mice and rabbits, tRNA genes of yeast and ribosomal genes of Drosophila.***

β-globin Gene: Haemoglobin consists of two α and β polypeptide chains. One of the β-chains is made up of 146 amino acid residues. The gene which codes for this polypeptide chain is called the β-globin gene. The precursor RNA of mouse β-globin gene has two intervening sequences, one 550 nucleotides long and the other 125 nucleotides long, which are excised during processing to form mRNA. Thus about two-thirds of the gene is discarded during processing.

The nucleotide sequences of three of the eight yeast tyrosine-tRNA genes have been determined. Each gene has a 14-base (ATTTAYCAC TACGA) intervening sequence in the middle. Similarly phe-tRNA genes have intervening sequences of 18-19 base pairs. It is noteworthy that in all the tRNA gene sequences the intervening sequences are adjacent to the anticodon triplet.

The discovery of split genes has *disturbed the concept of colinearity of genes,* according to which there is an almost exact correspondence between the nucleotide sequence and the amino acid sequence which it specifies. The presence of intervening sequences which do not take part in polypeptide chain formation goes against the colinearity concept.

There can no longer be exact correspondence between gene codons and amino acids. The discovery of several examples of split genes in eukaryotes indicates that colinearity between genes and their products may be an exception rather than a rule.

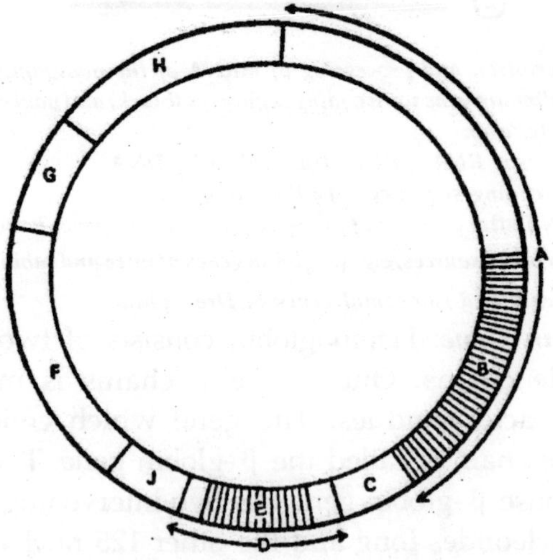

Genetic map of the bacteriophage ϕ X 174. Note the overlapping of gene E over gene D and of gene B over gene A.

Overlapping Genes

Genes within Genes: According to one of the dogmas of the genetic code each gene is responsible for the coding of one protein/polypeptide. This hypothesis was proposed by Beadle and Tatum in the 1940s and is called the one gene, one protein hypothesis. Barrell and his co-workers (1976) first gave evidence that suggests the possibility of overlapping of genes in the bacterial virus ϕ X174.

The bacteriophage consists of an icosahedral protein capsid containing single-stranded circular DNA. Genetic mapping techniques have shown that the bacteriophage has 9 genes (arranged in the order A-B-C-D-E-J-F-G-H) which code for 9 proteins.

The functions of these genes are as follows:

Gene A	–	DNA replication.
Genes B and D	–	assembly of phage particle,
Gene C	–	function not known.
Genes F, G and H	–	for structural capsid proteins. Barrell *et al* presented evidence that the proteins coded by Genes D and E are specified by the same segment of DNA.

The genetic code assumes the coding of each amino acid unit of the protein molecule by a *codon* of three nucleotides (triplet). In almost all organisms the total length of the DNA molecule available for coding proteins exceeds the total length of the protein product. In the phage ϕ X174, however, the total length of the proteins coded is more than the length of the DNA coding it.

Sanger and his colleagues (1976, 1977) have mapped the entire nucleotide sequence of ϕ X174 DNA and phage G4 DNA. ϕ X174 DNA contains 5,386 nucleotides. On the basis of the triplet code this number should code for a maximum of about 1,800 amino acids having a total weight of about

200,000 daltons. Actually, however, the total proteins coded have a molecular weight of 250,000 daltons. The phage DNA which should have a coding capacity of 5 to 6 average-sized protein molecules actually codes for 9 proteins. The virus DNA is thus apparently 10 to 15% too short for the total proteins coded.

A comparison of the DNA base sequence with the amino acid sequences of the proteins coded revealed that in two cases the same gene coded for two different proteins. Thus two genes which should normally have coded two proteins actually coded four. Sanger and his co workers found that gene B (360 nucleotides) was completely contained within gene A (1536 nucleotides). Similarly, gene E (273 nucleotides) was contained in gene D (1456 nucleotides).

The protein synthesised by gene B is not simply a shorter version of that synthesised by gene A. The two proteins have completely different amino acid sequences. Similarly with the proteins synthesised by genes D and E. It has been explained that the coding of two proteins by one gene is achieved by a shift in frame reading. For example, a reading frame of..........G, AAG, TTA, ACA.......... nucleotides codes for the amino acids *lysine, leucine* and *threonine*.

If the frame is read from one point earlier it becomes GAA, GTT, AAC, A....which codes for *glutamine, valine* and *asparagine*. Thus, the same gene can code for two different sequences by a frame shift (overlapping code) and produce two totally different proteins. Since one gene codes for more than one protein an amendment to the one-gene, one-protein dogma becomes necessary, at least in a few cases like ϕX174 and G4.

Another interesting fact is that the *termination codon* of gene D and the *initiation codon* of gene J overlap by one nucleotide: ---T–A–AT–G---

Termination Codon of Gene D. Initiation Codon of Gene J.

The bacteriophage G4 which infects *E. coli* also has overlapping genes. Gene B is completely contained within gene A and gene E within gene D (Fig.). Gene K is made up of the last 86 nucleotides of gene A and the first 89 nucleotides of gene C.

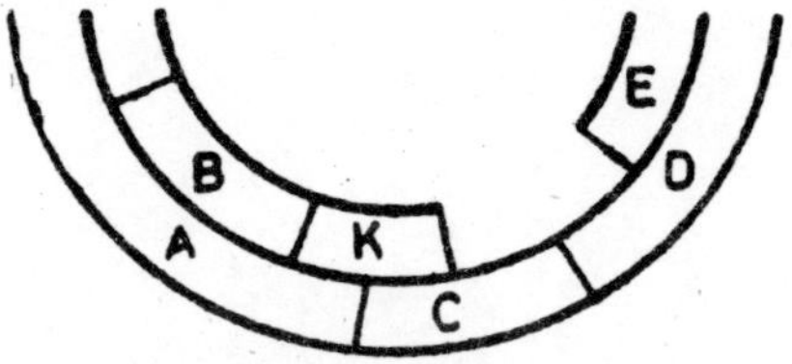

A part of the genetic map of the virus G4 showing overlapping genes.

The condition of overlapping genes is not of common occurrence. It may have arisen in the smaller viruses because of the limitations of the quantity of DNA that can be enclosed in the small viral capsides.

9

The Gametes

Germ cells and their involvement in fertilization or parthenogenesis provide continuity of life between generations. In many animals (e.g. insects, roundworms and vertebrates), there is an early separation of germ cells from somatic cells. In other animals and in almost all plant systems, such an early separation does not exist and from a seemingly similar type of cells derived from the zygote, germ cells are subsequently, differentiated. In plants also, from a vegetative apical meristem, floral meristems are differentiated, which develop flowers bearing the germ cells. It has also been shown that in animals, where the germ line separates early, the germ cells do not originate within the gonads, but instead their precursors called primordial germ cells (PGCs) migrate into the developing gonads.

The germ cells, once produced in whatever manner, take part in reproduction. The male and female gametes fuse together during fertilization, giving rise to a zygote, which develops into a complete organism. However, in many instances, both in animals and plants, the fertilization does not occur and the female gamete develops directly into a complete organism through a phenomenon described as parthenogenesis. Since the fusion of gametes to form a zygote is often described as amphimixis, the development of an entire organism without the fusion of two types of gametes is described as apomixis, a term more often used in plant systems. Parthenogenetic development of egg in certain animals and apomixis in certain plants are regular methods of reproduction and serve useful purposes. In this chapter, we propose to discuss the various aspects of sexual reproduction in animals and plants, including production of gametes and their participation in the development of whole organisms with or without the event of fertilization.

Reprodution in Animal Systems

Germ Cell Determination by Chromosome Diminution: Nematode—*Parascaris aequorum:* Germ cell determination in a roundworm, *Parascaris aequorum* (formerly *Ascaris megalocephala)* is dependent on the distribution of the germplasm (a part of the cytoplasm) in the zygote. This nematode has only two chromosomes per haploid cell ($n = 2$). The first division of the zygote gives two cells, one of them having chromosomes which undergo fragmentation and the other with the germplasm having intact chromosomes. The fragmented chromosomes lead to loss of numerous genes. At four-celled stage also, three cells undergo chromosome diminution (Fig.).

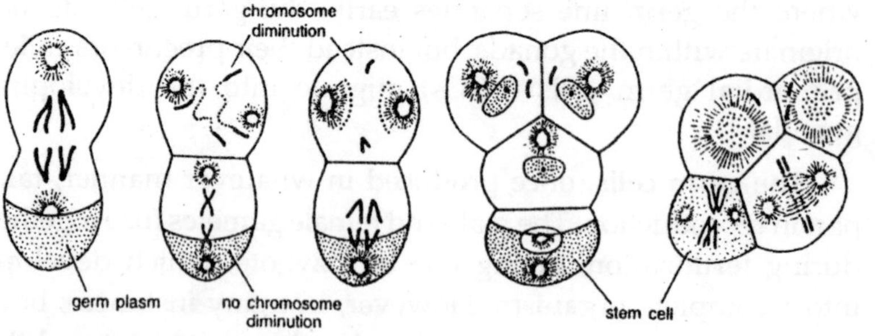

(a) normal zygote undergoing chromosome diminution during cleavage

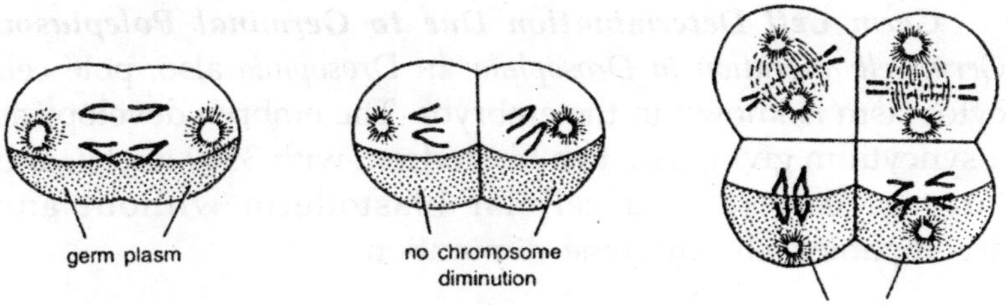

(b) centrifuged zygote undergoing no chromosome diminution during cleavage

Distribution of germplasm during cleavage in Parascaris showing chromosomal diminution in three cells developing into somatic cells and lack of chromosomal diminution in one stem cell, which develops into germ cells (redrawn from Glbert, Developmental Biology, 1994).

At 16-celled stage, only two cells have undiminished chromosomes, one of them developing into germ cells and the other again undergoing chromosome diminution forming somatic cells. Thus the cells retaining complete set of intact chromosomes form the germ cells and those undergoing chromosome diminution form the somatic cells. It is obvious that one of the two poles of the zygote, called vegetal end had cytoplasm containing factors that protect nuclei from chromosomal diminution giving rise to germ cells.

The Midge (Wachtiella persicariae): In the midge, *Wachtiella persicariae,* most nuclei of the early embryo lose 32 of their original 40 chromosomes, but two nuclei at the posterior pole of the egg do not divide for sometime, and eventually give rise to germ cells. If none of the nuclei is allowed to migrate into the posterior pole region by ligation, every nucleus undergoes diminution and no germ cells are formed, so that the midge is sterile. It has been shown that the germinal cytoplasm or germplasm at one pole is different and carried factors protecting nuclei from chromosome diminution. If this germinal cytoplasm was removed or destroyed by ultraviolet irradiation, it gave sterile individuals. This posterior poleplasm or germinal cytoplasm is marked with polar granules facilitating its identification, although the causal relationship of polar granules with germ cell determination is not established.

Germ Cell Determination Due to Germinal Poleplasm: *Germ cell migration in Drosophila:* In *Drosophila* also, pole cell cytoplasm is known in the embryos. The embryo develops as a syncytium giving rise to a blastoderm with 3500 nuclei, and later gives rise to a cellular blastoderm without any accompanied chromosome diminution.

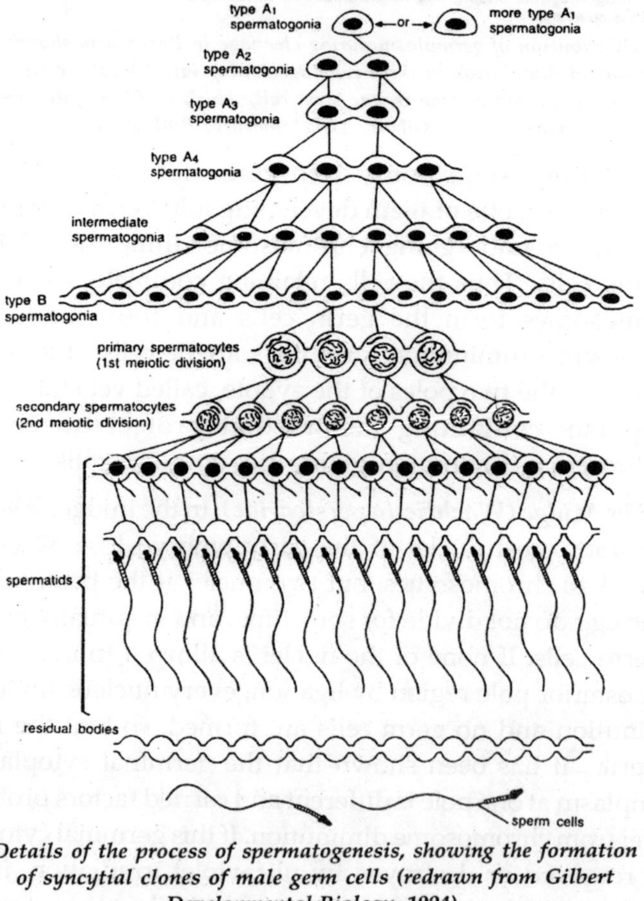

Details of the process of spermatogenesis, showing the formation of syncytial clones of male germ cells (redrawn from Gilbert Developmental Biology, 1994).

Further fate of the cells of the blastoderm depends on the region of the embryo to which these cells or nuclei migrate. It has been shown that a small amount of anucleate poleplasm at the posterior end is responsible for determination of germ cells, so that if this poleplasm is transferred to anterior end of another embryo, the anterior pole will give rise to germ cell precursors. This suggests that the poleplasm is directly concerned with germ cell determination.

Germinal Poleplasm in Amphibians: In frog eggs also, the vegetal region of the fertilized egg contains material similar to that present in the poleplasm of *Drosophila*. This germinal cytoplasm was found in few cells of presumptive ectoderm; these few cells are the primordial germ cells precursors. Therefore, like the poleplasm of *Drosophila*, the cytoplasm from the vegetal region of frog zygotes contains the determinants for germ cell formation.

The Gametogenesis: The separation of somatic cells and germ cells is one of the first events of cell differentiation to occur during animal development. In animal systems, the germ cells eventually migrate to the gonads, where they differentiate into gametes, a phenomenon called gametogenesis.

Spermatogenesis: Spermatogenesis is the process by which 'primordial germ cells' generate sperms through meiotic divisions. The primary spermatocytes which undergo meiosis, are formed after the primordial germ cells have undergone various stages of development and several cycles of cell division. During embryo development, the germ cells arrive at the genital ridge of male embryo and get incorporated into the sex cords, become hollow to form 'seminiferous tubules', and the epithelium of these tubules differentiate into the Sertoli cells. On the surface of spermatogenic cells as well as Sertoli cells are present N-cadherin molecules. In addition, on the surface of spermatogenic cells are also present galactosyltransferase molecules which bind with their receptors on Sertoli cells. Thus the N-cadherins as well as the galactosyltransferase receptor system help spermatogenic cells to bind to the Sertoli cells. Spermatogenesis really occurs in the recesses of the Sertoli cells, which nourish and protect the development of sperm cells.

The details of the process of spermatogenesis has been studied in several organisms, but we like to discuss only those in mammals. In mammals, the PGCs, after reaching the gonad divide to form type A_1 spermatogonia, which divide each to form another type A_1 spermatogoniun and a type A_2 spermatogonium. The type A_2 spermatogonia divide to form A_3 spermatogonia, which form A_4 spermatogonia, and finally the' intermediate spermatogonia (which are committed to become spermatozoa). Intermediate spermatogonia divide by a mitotic division to form type B spermatogonia, each dividing again by a mitotic division to form primary spermatocytes, which by meiotic division first form secondary spermatocytes and then the haploid cells called spermatids. The spermatids differentiate into sperm cells (Fig.).

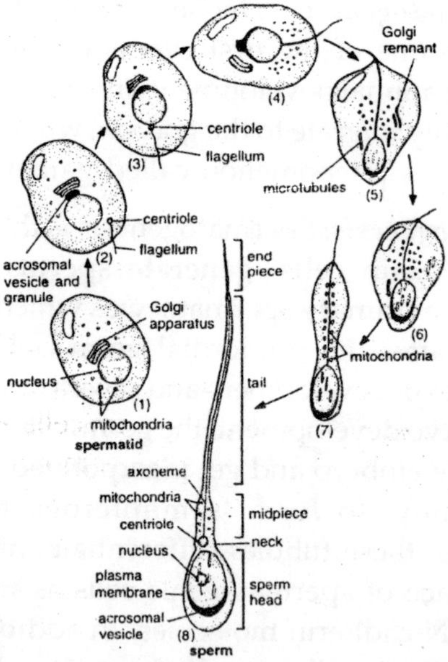

Modification of germ cell to form mammalian sperm. The centriole gives rise long flagellum and Golgi forms the acrosomal vesicle. The size of mature sperm is enlarged to show details (redrawn from Gilbert, Developmental Biology 1994).

During spermatogonial divisions, cytokinesis is not complete and cells remain connected through cytoplasmic bridges (l μ m in diameter), so that even haploid spermatids are functionally diploid having gene products from all the genes in a diploid.

The maturation of spermatids into sperm cells is called spermeogenesis (or spermateliosis). The sperm differentiation involves the following alterations in spermatid (Fig.):

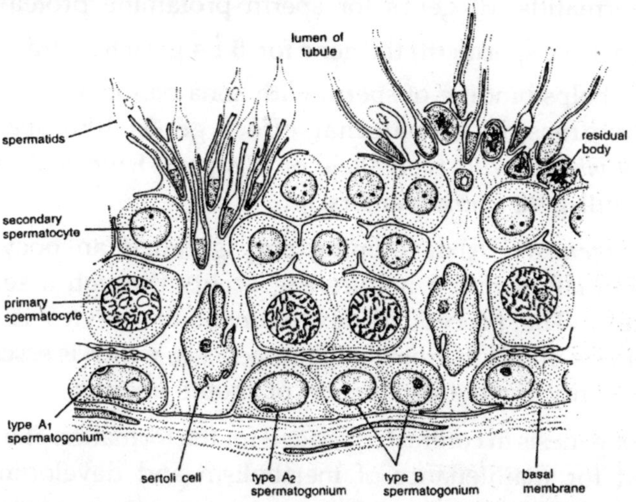

A section of the seminiferous tubule showing the relationship between sertoli cells and the developing sperm ; as cells mature, they move towards the lumen (redrawn from Gilbert Developmental Biology, 1994).

(i) construction of acrosomal vesicle from the Golgi apparatus; the acrosome forms a cap over the nucleus;

(ii) sperm nucleus rotates so that acrosome cap will now face the basal membrane of seminiferous tubule;

(iii) the centriole on the other side of the nucleus now forms the flagellum, which extends in the lumen (Fig.);

(iv) the nucleus flattens and condenses, and mitochondria form a ring around the base of the flagellum. The mature sperms then enter the lumen of seminiferous tubule.

During spermatogenesis, specific genes necessary for sperm motility or binding to the egg are expressed. Following genes are expressed during meiotic prophase: (i) Y chromosome specific genes; (ii) (β 2-tubulin gene (in *Drosophila)*, necessary for meiotic spindles and the axoneme; (iii) the gene for the protein, bindin. The following additional genes are expressed in spermatids: (i) genes for sperm protamine proteins that compact the sperm; (ii) the gene for β 1,4 galactosyltransferase which helps binding of sperm with zona pallucida of the egg; (iii) expression of paternal effect genes like *spe-11* in *Caenorhabditis*(wild type allele of this gene from male parent only will give normal embryo).

Oogenesis: A developing egg is called an oocyte. Its differentiation into a mature egg occurs through a series of changes. The process of development of oocytes is called oogenesis. It differs from spermatogenesis, which is essentially meant only for the production of motile sperms.

Oogenesis in contrast, is needed for the formation of oocytes, suited for maintenance of metabolism and development of embryo. Therefore the oocyte contains a complex cytoplasm with enzymes, mRNAs organelles and metabolic substrates (Table).

While in species like sea urchin, a female produces hundreds or thousands of eggs at a time, in other species like humans only a few eggs are produced during the whole lifetime of an individual.

Components Stored in Mature Oocyte of Xenopus Laevis

Component	*Excess over liver cells*
Mitochondria	100,000
RNA polymerases	60,000 to 100,000
DNA polymerases	100,000

Contd...

Component	*Excess over liver cells*
Ribosomes	200,000
tRNA	10,000
Histones	15,000
dNTPs (deoxyribo-nucleoside triphosphates)	2,500

The primordial germ cells (PGCs) migrate to developing gonads to become oogonia, and eventually differentiate into primary oocytes. In species like sea urchin, oogonia are self renewing stem cells, surviving throughout the life time. In humans, on the other hand, thousands of oogonia divide rapidly upto seventh month of gestation to form 7×10^6 germ cells, most of which die before birth and the remaining germ cells enter the first prophase of meiosis forming what are called the primary oocytes. These primary oocytes continue to die even after birth and only about 400 oocytes mature during the life time of a female. These reach diplotene and stay at this stage till puberty after which, periodically meiocytes undergo meiosis in groups.

The nucleus of an oocyte, called 'germinal vesicle', breaks down and the metaphase spindle migrates to the periphery of the cell. The resumption of meiosis in amphibians requires the hormone progesterone. The first division gives a secondary oocyte and the first polar body. In the second meiotic division, second polar body and the haploid egg are produced. The egg is released by the process of ovulation. This production of three polar bodies and an egg containing the entire cytoplasm of the oocyte is in sharp contrast of spermatogenesis, where four sperms with equal cytoplasm are produced.

In fishes and frogs, each year a new cohort of oocytes is produced and oocytes last for three years as in *Rana pipiens.*

In the first two years oocytes increase in size gradually and in the third year they swell to their characteristic size due to accumulation of yolk. The phase before this accumulation of yolk during prophase I is described as previtellogenic phase and the yolk forming phase is described as vitellogenic phase, which starts when oocytes reach diplotene as described above (Fig.).

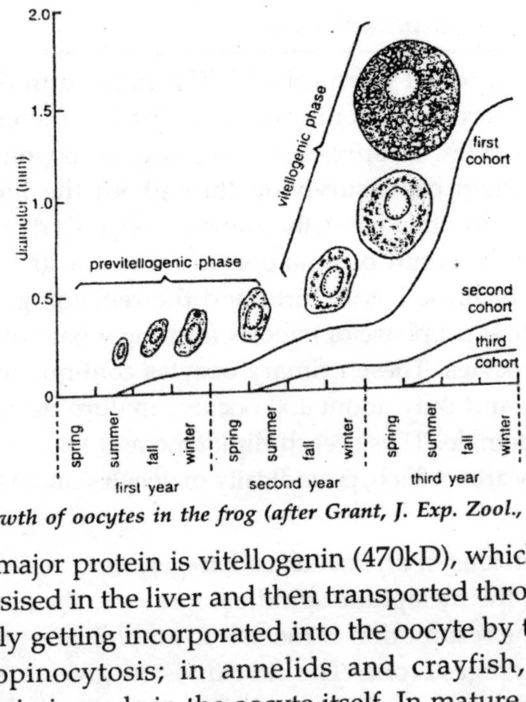

Growth of oocytes in the frog (after Grant, J. Exp. Zool., 1953).

The major protein is vitellogenin (470kD), which, in frogs, is synthesised in the liver and then transported through blood, eventually getting incorporated into the oocyte by the process of micropinocytosis; in annelids and crayfish, however, vitellogenin is made in the oocyte itself. In mature oocyte, the vitellogenin is split into heavily phosphorylated phosvitin and the lipoprotein Hipovitellin, both packaged into yolk platelets. The amount of yolk increases in the vegetal hemisphere, which eventually contains nearly 75% of the yolk. At this stage the glycogen granules, ribosomes, lipid vesicles, and ER are found towards the animal pole. The cortical granules, mitochondria and pigment granules are found at the periphery of the cell within the oocyte cortex. Each specific mRNA also becomes localised in certain regions of the oocyte. For instance Vgl mRNA and (β -globin mRNA are translocated to vegetal cortex.

Certain hormonal interactions regulate the events during leptotene and thereafter in the following order: (i) gonadotropin releasing hormone is secreted by hypothalamus and received by the pituitary; (ii) pituitary secretes gonadotropic hormones into the blood; (iii) the hormones stimulate the follicle cells to secrete oestrogen and progesterone; (iv) oestrogen induces the liver to synthesise and secrete vitellogenin; (v) progesterone stimulates meiosis (through the synthesis of C-mos protein), by the occurrence of germinal vesicle breakdown (GVBD).

Active gene transcription also takes place in the growing oocytes. Some details of relative rates of DNA synthesis, tRNA synthesis and rRNA synthesis during amphibian oogenesis are given in Figure.

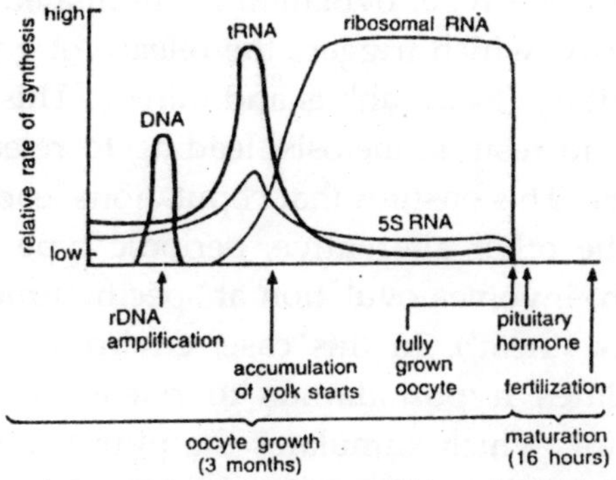

Relative rates of the synthesis of DNA, tRNA and rRNA during the last three months of amphibian oogenesis (redrawn from Gilbert Developmental Biology, 1994).

Oogenesis in Insects vs Mammals: Several types of oogenesis are known in insects but more details are known about what is called meroistic oogenesis in *Drosophila*. Each oogonium divides four times giving 16 cells called cystocytes which are connected to each other by ring canals. Only one of these cells forms an oocyte, other 15 cells become nurse cells (Fig.). The RNA synthesis is largely confined to these nurse cells (chromosomes become polytenic in these cells), and RNA made by these cells is transported to oocyte cytoplasm.

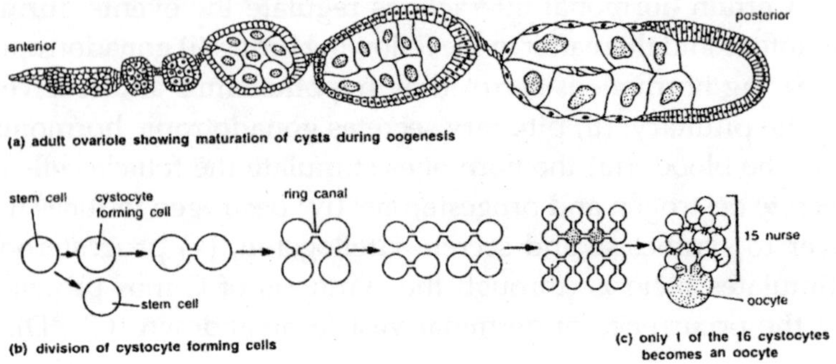

The formation of 16 interconnected cystocytes in Drosophila, and the development of only one of these 16 cystocytes into an oocyte (redrawn from Gilbert Developmental Biology, 1994).

In mammals, oogenesis follows one of the two basic patterns: (i) In one type, ovulation is stimulated by physical intercourse only, which triggers the release of gonadotropins from the pituitary (as in rabbits and minks). This gives signal to the oocyte to resume meiosis, leading to release of ovum from the ovary. This ensures that copulations lead to fertilized ova. (ii) In the other alternative, periodic type of ovulation occurs, which, involves ovulation at specific time of the year called oestrus ('heat'). In this case, environment (heat and light) stimulates hypothalamus to release gonadotropin-releasing factor, which stimulates the pituitary to release its gonadotropins (follicle-stimulating hormone, or FSH and the luteinizing hormone or LH), which induce follicle cells to proliferate and secrete oestrogen. This evokes the pattern of-mating behaviour characteristic of the species, and causes ovulation to occur.

In humans also, periodic ovulation occurs, each cycle being 29.5 days, but no yearly oestrus or 'heat' occurs. The majority of oocytes are maintained in the prolonged diplotene stage (often referred to as the dictyate stage). The oocyte . undergoes 500-fold increase in volume (diameter increases from 10 μ m to

80 μ m), with increased number of follicular granulosa cells around it, forming cumulus. A cavity called antrum is also formed during the growth of the follicle and gets filled with a mixture of proteins, hormones, cAMP and other molecules.

Format of Gametes

The Sperm: Each sperm is known to consist of a haploid nucleus, a propulsion system to move the nucleus and a sac of enzymes that enable the nucleus to enter the egg. Most of the cytoplasm of the sperm cell is exhausted during maturation of the sperm, which on maturity contains only some organelles suitably modified to perform special function. A mature sperm consists of: (i) sperm head, (ii) neck, (iii) midpiece, (iv) tail, and (v) end piece (Fig.). The sperm head contains a nucleus, which becomes streamlined with tightly compressed DNA and an acrosomal vesicle. The acrosomal vesicle is derived from the Golgi apparatus and contains several enzymes, that digest proteins and complex sugars, when the sperm enters the egg. The acrosomal vesicle can thus be compared with a lysosome.

The sperm is propelled with the help of a flagellum, but in some cases (e.g. *Ascaris),* it travels by amoeboid motion of lamellipodia formed due to local extensions of the cell membrane. Flagella themselves are complex structures each consisting of an axoneme formed of microtubules extending from the centriole at the base of the nucleus.

The Egg (ovum): Unlike sperm (which eliminates cytoplasm during maturation), the egg retains most of its cytoplasm which is needed for the beginning of growth and development. The egg also synthesises and absorbs proteins such as yolk that works as food reserve for the developing embryo. Consequently the egg may attain a size ($22 \times 10^5/\mu m$) as much as 10,000 times the volume of the sperm (Fig.). The stored material in the egg includes proteins, ribosomes, tRNAs, mRNA and morphogenetic factors for growth and development. The proteins are needed for supply of energy in early embryonic cells. The ribosomes, tRNAs and mRNA (as many as 2500-5000 types of mRNAs are found in a sea urchin egg) are needed for active protein synthesis soon after fertilization (the mRNA molecules remain dormant until after fertilization). The morphogenetic factors, localised in different regions of the egg, direct the differentiation of cells into certain cell types during, early cell divisions.

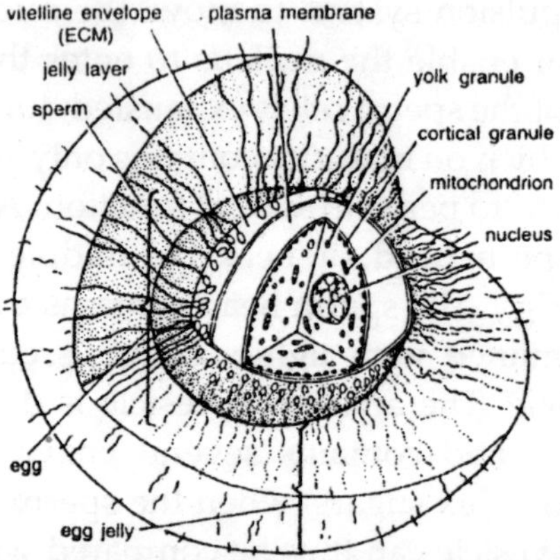

Structure of sea urchin egg during fertilization (redrawn from Gilbert Developmental Biology, 1994).

The outermost layer of the egg is the vitelline membrane followed by the plasma membrane, which regulates the transport of ions during fertilization and facilitates fusion with the sperm plasma membrane (many types of eggs also have an egg jelly outside the vitelline envelope; this may attract sperms). The vitelline membrane remains adhered to the plasma membrane with the help of extensions from the plasma membrane and is essential for species-specific binding of sperm. In mammalian egg, the vitelline envelope is a thick extracellular matrix (ECM) called zona pallucida surrounded by a layer of cells called cumulus cells, which represent ovarian follicular cells nurturing the egg at the time of its release from the ovary.

On the inner side of plasma membrane, in the egg lies the cortex, which is more gel like than the cytoplasm and contains high concentration of globular actin molecules forming microfilaments during fertilization.

The microfilaments are needed for cell division and for extension of egg surface into microvilli, which help sperm entry into the egg cell. The cortex contains cortical granules derived from Golgi apparatus and is thus comparable to acrosomal vesicle of the sperm.

There can be as many as 15,000 cortical granules in an egg as compared to one acrosomal vesicle in a sperm. These granules contain digestive enzymes, mucopolysaccharides, adhesive glycoproteins and hyaline protein. The enzymes and mucopolysaccharides prevent further entry of sperm after the first sperm has entered. The adhesive glycoproteins and the hyaline proteins surround early embryo to provide support for early blastomeres.

Recognition of Egg and Sperm

Sperm Attraction and Activation from a Distance: In many animal systems (e.g. cnidarians, molluscs, echinoderms and urochordates), it has been conclusively shown that there is species specific attraction of sperms towards the egg (this attraction is not always species specific). In some cases, even the timing of this attraction was found to depend on a particular stage of egg development. This attraction seems to depend on the release of a chemotactic factor from the egg (the oocyte). One such chemotactic molecule characterised in sea urchin is called 'resact', a 14 amino acid peptide, which attracts sperms of one species and not those of the other species.

When the sperm comes in contact of the egg jelly or the egg surface, the sperm gets activated (in sea urchin, it is due to a sulfated polysaccharide) leading to an acrosome reaction having following two components: (i) in the first part of the reaction, the acrosomal vesicle of the sperm head fuses with the sperm plasma membrane and releases its contents (digestive enzymes); (ii) the second part of acrosome reaction involves extension of the acrosome process due to polymerisation of globular actin molecules forming actin filaments. This is facilitated by the release of hydrogen ions from the sperm head. The increase in pH due to release of hydrogen ions also activates the dynein ATPase in the neck of the sperm, and leads to increase in mitochondrial respiration. The energy released from ATP and respiration is used for flagellar motility. The details of the steps involved in acrosome reaction in sea urachin are shown in.

Recognition by Contact of Gametes (sea urchin): In sea urchin, once the acrosomal process (formed as above) penetrates the egg jelly, it comes in contact of the vitelline envelope, where species specific recognition takes place. This species specific recognition is mediated by the protein 'bindin' located on the acrosomal process exactly at the point where it should be for sperm-egg recognition.

It has been shown that 'bindins' of even closely related species differ, since species-specific bindin receptors are found on the vitelline envelope. The bindin receptor is a trans-membrane glycoprotein of 1300 amino acids, its binding region projecting in the extracellular space, thus becoming a component of vitelline envelope. Hundreds of these receptor molecules are needed for adhesion of a sperm to the egg surface.

Contact of Sperm and Egg (mouse): In mammals; zona pallucida plays the same role as vitelline envelope in sea urchin. Zona pallucida (a glycoprotein matrix secreted by growing oocyte) thus binds the sperm. Of the three glycoproteins (ZP1, ZP2, ZP3) isolated from zona pallucida, ZP3 (83kD) is the only glycoprotein, which is competitive for sperm binding and acts as sperm receptor. A set of proteins on the sperm are capable of recognizing a specific carbohydrated protein region of ZP3 present on zona pallucida of the egg. After approaching the egg, the sperm does not really penetrate, but rather wriggles on the egg surface.

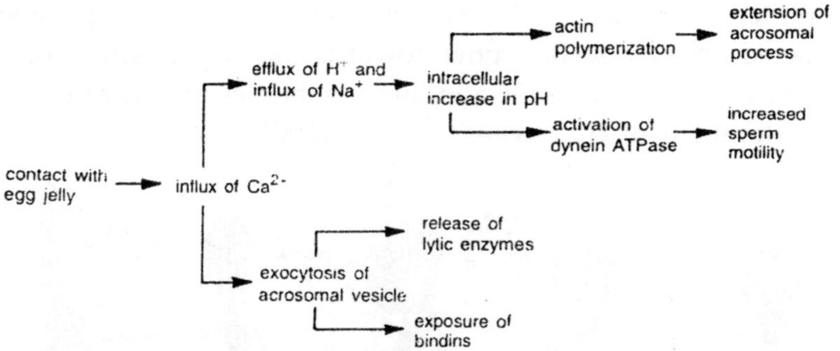

Interrelationships in the process of acrosome reaction in sea urchin (redrawn from Gilbert Developmental Biology, 1994).

This wriggling is facilitated by three proteins on the sperm surface; (i) a 56 kD peptide exposed on the sperm membrane, that binds to the galactose residues of ZP3, thus working as a receptor for ZP3; (ii) a 60 kD glycosyltransferase enzyme on sperm cell membrane, that recognises the sugar N-acetylglucosamine on ZP3, but can not catalyze it for want of a second necessary reactant; (iii) a 95 kD transmembrane protein with an extracellular site that facilitates binding with ZP3, and an intracellular site that has a tyrosine kinase enzyme activity involved in phosphorylation of intracellular enzymes after the protein binds to ZP3.

After the binding of a sperm with ZP3 of the egg, the acrosome reaction (release of enzymes from acrosomai vesicle and extension of acrosomai process) is initiated in mammals like mouse. This reaction is induced by ZP3 glycoproteins, and the tyrosine kinase (95 kD) of ZP3 receptor plays an important role in this reaction.

During the acrosome reaction, the anterior portion of the sperm plasma membrane carrying ZP3 binding proteins is shed, although sperm still remains attached (by secondary binding facilitated by proteins like ZP2 or proacrosine in the inner acrosomai membrane) to find a path into the interior of the egg (Fig.). After a mouse sperm enters the egg, the contents of the egg's cortical granules are released. These contents contain a protease that alters ZP2 in such a manner, that other acrosome reacted sperms do not move towards the egg. A study of a number of these proteins and their antibodies may lead to the development of contraceptives for humans.

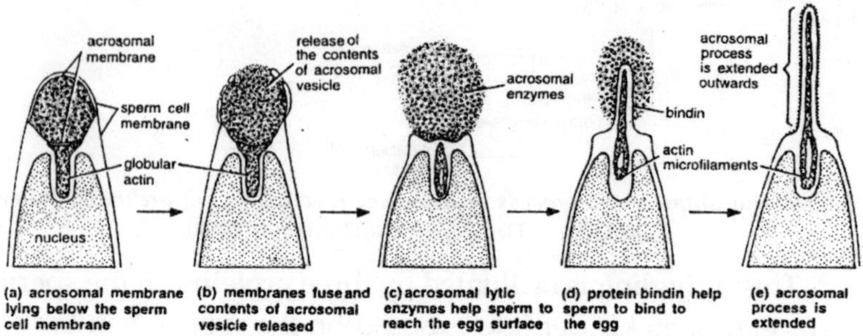

Acrosome reactions in echinoderm sperm (redrawn from Gilbert Developmental Biology, 1994).

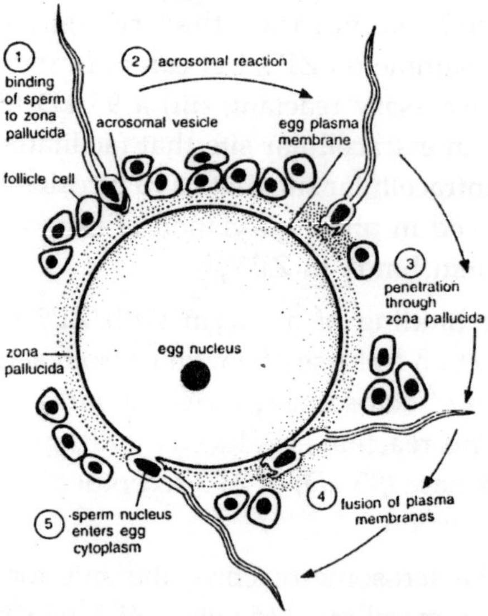

The acrosomai reaction, when mammalian sperm fertilizes an egg (redrawn from Alberts et al. Molecular Biology of the Cell, 1994).

Egg-sperm Membrane Fusion and Prevention of Polyspermy: After sperm-egg contact, the vitelline envelope or zona pallicida releases its contents at the point of contact leading to fusion of sperm. It causes the polymerisation of actin and the extension of several microvilli to form the fertilization cone comparable to acrosome process in sperm. The fusion of membranes also leads to the formation of a cytoplasmic bridge through which the sperm nucleus and the tail pass to the egg interior. This fusion is an active process facilitated by specific fusogenic proteins (*e.g.*, HA protein of influenza virus, F protein of Sendal virus and bindin of mouse).

Since polyspermy due to the entry of more than one sperms into an egg can be disastrous, there are mechanisms, which prevent entry of more than one sperm into the egg. In sea urchin, there are two such mechanisms:

(i) a fast reaction involving an electrical charge in plasma membrane and

(ii) slower reaction involving exocytosis of cortical granules. The ionic concentration (Na^+, K^+) of the egg is very different from its surroundings, the Na^+ concentration being low and K^+ concentration being high. The resting membrane potential is generally about 70 millivolts (-70mV, inside being negatively charged), at which sperm can fuse with egg membrane. Within 1-3 seconds after the binding of sperm, this potential shifts to a positive level (20mV), at which sperm and egg membranes can not fuse. The shift occurs due to opening of sodium channels which allow entry of Na^+ ions into the egg changing the membrane potential. The opening of sodium channel has been shown to be dependent on an acrosomal protein, which presumably gets activated due to binding of the sperm to the egg.

In sea urchin, the fast block to polyspermy due to shift in membrane potential is transient, and persists only for a minute. Subsequently, the sperms bound to vitelline membrane are removed with the help of cortical granules released from the egg.

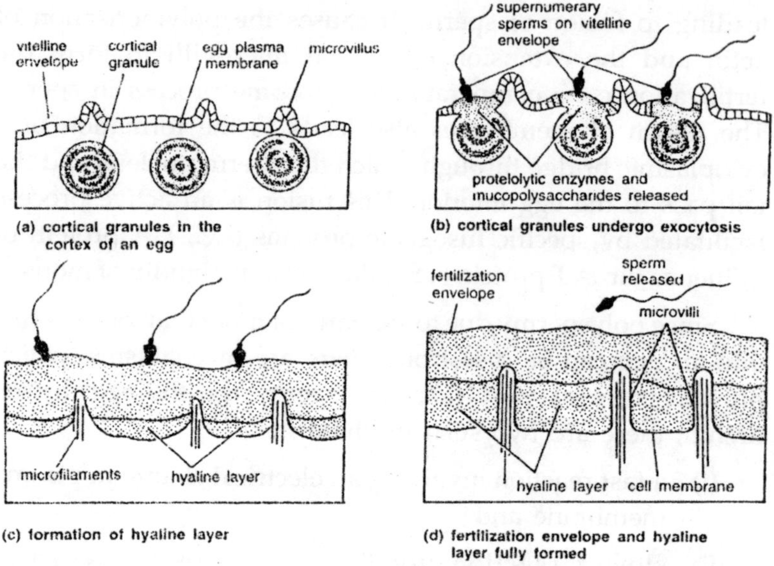

Cortical granule exocytosis, showing the events leading to the formation of the fertilization envelope and the hyaline layer (redrawn from Gilbert, Developmental Biology, 1994).

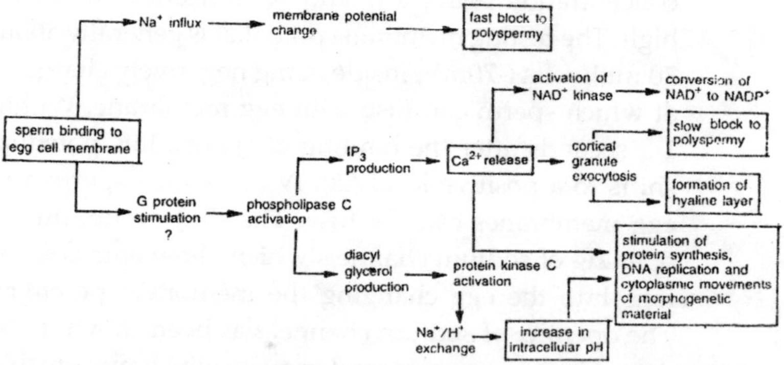

Different steps of sea urchin egg metabolism activated by sperm binding and entry into the egg (redrawn from Gilbert, Developmental Biology 1994).

In each egg there are about 15,000 such granules, which fuse with-egg plasma membrane and release their contents soon after the entry of a sperm. This exocytosis and the entire cortical reaction is associated with elevated concentration of calcium ions (Ca^{2+}) followed by the release of these calcium ions. Several proteins which facilitate exocytosis of cortical granules, include proteases, which help in removing the bindin protein and sperms attached to the vitelline envelope. Mucopolysaccharides, also released from cortical granules, produce an osmotic gradient causing water to rush in the space between vitelline envelope and cell membrane, so that the vitelline envelope expands and becomes fertilization envelope (Fig.). A peroxidase hardens this fertilization envelope and another protein hyalin forms a coating around the egg.

In mammals, instead of the formation of a fertilization envelope, zona pallucida receptors get so modified that they can no longer allow binding of sperms. This modification is described as 'zona reaction', during which ZP3 and ZP2 get modified so that the sperm can no longer initiate or maintain its binding to the zona pallucida.

Egg Metabolism During Fertilization: In sea urchin, the egg is metabolically sluggish but becomes active by the entry of the sperm. The sperm entry sets in motion a pre-pogrammed set of events shown in Figure. As shown in Figure and summarised in Table, following events (increase in pH, increase in Ca^{++} and decrease in Na^{+} and H^{+}) are involved in the metabolic activity that accompanies the different steps in fertilization. Sodium influx and intracellular release of calcium leading to decrease in Na^{+} and increase of Ca^{++} in the cytoplasm, thus block polyspermy.

The intracellular release of Ca^{++} activates the following metabolic reactions: (i) activation of NAD^{+} kinase converting NAD^{+} to $NADP^{+}$ for lipid biosynthesis required for cell membrane formation during cleavage; (ii) oxygen consumption in respiration leading to reduction in O_2 concentration, required to cross-link the fertilization membrane; (iii) influx of Na^{+} and eflux of H^{+} leading to increase in pH from 6.8 to 7.2; this leads to activation of DNA synthesis and protein synthesis utilizing mRNA already present in the egg, thus helping in the fusion of gametes.

Rearrangement of Egg Cytoplasm after Fertilization: The cytoplasm of the egg contains morphogenetic determinants, which get distributed to the different and specific regions of the cell due to rearrangement of the cytoplasm. This distribution of morphogenetic determinants due to rearrangement of cytoplasm is crucial for cell differentiation later in the development.

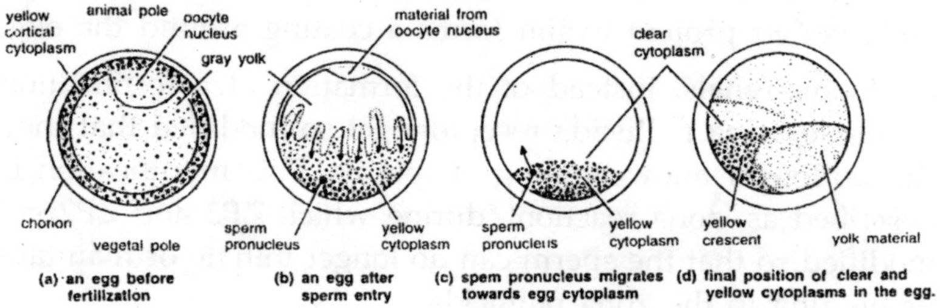

Cytoplasmic rearrangement in the egg of the tunicate Styela partita (redrawn from Gilbert, Developmental Biology, 1994).

The rearrangement of cytoplasm of the egg has been studied in the tunicate *Styela partita.* The egg in this animal consists of gray cytoplasm enveloped by a cortical layer. During meiosis the nucleus breaks down and releases a substance that accumulates in the animal (upper) hemisphere of the egg. After entry of sperm, within 5 minutes the inner clear and cortical yellow cytoplasm migrates into the vegetal (lower) hemisphere. The male pronucleus and the lipid inclusions move from vegetal pole to the equator along the future posterior side of the embryo. This leads to the formation of a yellow crescent.

The rearrangement of cytoplasm in the egg has also been observed in frog. After entry of the sperm, the cortical (outer) cytoplasm shifts about 30° towards the point of sperm entry relative to the inner cytoplasm. This leads to the formation of a region called gray crescent, which marks the region, where gastrulation is initiated. (Gray crescent is not found in all frogs; it is found in *Rana,* but not in *Xenopus;* however the rotation of cytoplasm takes place even in *Xenopus).* The movement of cytoplasm is facilitated by microtubules and motor proteins. The above rearrangements of egg cytoplasm initiate a cascade of events that determine the dorsal-ventral axis of the frog.

Fusion of the Genetic Material: The duration of the process of the nuclear fusion between sperm and egg varies from 1 hour in sea urchin to 12 hours in a mammal. The sperm enters the egg either perpendicular (sea urchin) or tangentially (mammals) to the egg surface.

After entry of sperm, the sperm nucleus and the. centrosome separate from its mitochondria and flagella, both of which soon undergo degeneration. Therefore, in the zygote, the nuclear genome is derived from both sperm and egg, the mitochondria are derived only from the egg and the centrosome is derived from the sperm only.

The egg nucleus, when haploid is called female pronucleus. The sperm nucleus after its entry in the egg cytoplasm, undergoes decondensation to form what is called male pronucleus. The decondensation of the sperm nucleus is facilitated by exchange of sperm nuclear proteins by those from the egg cytoplasm.

The decondensation starts with phosphorylation of two sperm specific histones (X,Y) bound tightly to DNA. The phosphorylation is brought about by the activation of cAMP dependent kinase induced by the contact of sperm with a sulphate rich compound in the egg jelly.

The phosphorylation, thus brought about, interferes with the binding of the histones X and Y with DNA. This leads to the loosening of these histones which are then replaced by H2A and H2B. This is facilitated by nucleoplasmin, to which though H2A and H2B remain bound, but which has greater affinity for the above sperm specific proteins X and Y. This restores nucleosome structure of sperm DNA (Fig.).

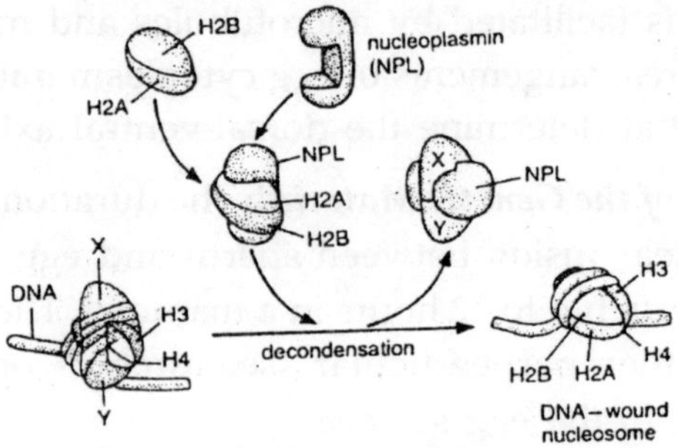

Remodelling of sperm chromatin during decondensation (redrawn from Gilbert Developmental Biology, 1994).

Some Characteristics of Fertilization in Sea Urchin and Mammals

		Sea urchin	*Mammal*
1.	Duration of nuclear fusion	4 hour	12 hours
2.	Entry of sperm	Perpendicular to the egg surface	Tangentially to the egg surface
3.	Fusion of nuclei	Fusion occurs giving a zygote	No fusion occurs, but chromosomes orient on a mitotic spindle producing two diploid nuclei

Events of Sea Urchin Fertilization

Event	*Approximate duration after sperm entry*
1. Sperm-egg binding	0 seconds
2. Fast block to polyspermy	< 3 seconds
3. Sperm-egg membrane fusion	< 30 seconds
4. Calcium increase starts	30 seconds
5. Cortical granule exocytosis (slow block to polyspermy)	30-60 seconds
6. Activation of NAD kinase,	

Contd...

Event		*Approximate duration after sperm entry*
	increase in NADH & NADPH & increase in O_2 consumption	Starts at 60 seconds
7.	Sperm entry	1-2 min
8.	Acid efflux and increase in pH	1-5 min
9.	Decondensation of sperm chromatin and migration of sperm nucleus to egg centre	2-12 min
10.	Migration of egg nucleus towards sperm nucleus	5-10 min
11.	Activation of protein synthesis & amino acid transport	Starts at 5-10 min
12.	Initiation of DNA synthesis	20-40 min
13.	Mitosis	60-80 min
14.	First cleavage	85-95 min

In sea urchin, after the sperm enters the egg, the male pronucleus rotates 180°, thus bringing the sperm centriole between the egg and the sperm pronuclei. The microtubules of the centriole from male nucleus extend towards the egg and two pronuclei migrate towards each other and fuse to form the zygote nucleus. The DNA synthesis starts in the zygote nucleus either before this fusion of the pronuclei or soon after fusion. The different events during fusion and their approximate duration in sea urchin and mammals are given in Tables.

In mammals, the female pronucleus enlarges, and oocyte completes second meiotic division. The two pronuclei replicate their DNA during their journey towards each other. On meeting, they break down their envelopes. No fusion occurs, but chromosomes from sperm and egg orient on a mitotic spindle producing two diploid nuclei rather than a zygote. A true diploid nucleus in mammals is first seen not in the zygote, but at the two cell stage.

Non-equivalence of Mammalian Pronuclei: Although, one of the basis of Mendelian genetics is the assumptions that male and female nuclei make equal contributions to the zygote, there is recent evidence that, in mammals they functionally differ and complement each other. It has been shown that certain developmentally active genes from the sperm and other developmentally active genes from the egg complement in the zygote for the development of the embryo, so that paternal and maternal pronuclei both are necessary for the development of mammalian embryo.

The Parthenogenesis: Partheogenesis is the development of egg without fertilization, and the adult animals developing through parthenogenesis are called parthenogenetic or parthenogenone or parthenote. However, such a development may still need activation of egg by a sperm.

Conditions intermediate between parthenogenesis and fertlization may also exist and include the following: (i) partial fertlization (where only a part of a sperm is involved in fertilization, e.g. in sea urchin); (ii) gynogenesis (where sperm enters the egg but degenerates without taking part in fertlization e.g. in *Rhabdites);* (iii) androgenesis (where the egg is activated by the sperm, but the egg nucleus does not take part in the development; instead egg with sperm nucleus develops in a paternal embryo, as observed in irradiated frog eggs); (iv) merogony (where, only a fragment of the egg fuses with the sperm and then develops in an embryo, as observed when eggs of sea urchin are shaken into pieces before being subjected to fertilization).

The significance of parthenogenesis lies in the fact that it provides a means for rapid breeding in aphids during the summer, when vegetation is abundant to feed on, and no male partners are needed for mating. In honey bees, it also helps in controlling the sex ratio.

Parthenogenesis may be diploid parthenogenesis (also

called thelytoky) or haploid parthenogenesis (also called arrehnotoky).

Diploid Parthenogenesis (thelytoky): In a few animal species, the female gametes are unreduced diploid and need not be fertilized for the restoration of its diploid chromosome number. Following are some variants of the mechanisms involved in the production of diploid egg: (i) One of the polar body may fuse with the oocyte giving diploid egg. (ii) In some insects (such as *Moraba virgo,* and the lizard *Cnemidophorus uniparens),* the oogonia double their chromosome number before meiosis; (iii) In grasshopper *Pycnoscelus surinamensis,* no meiosis takes place and the germ cells form diploid ova by two mitotic divisions. The diploid parthenogenesis can be obligatory or cyclical.

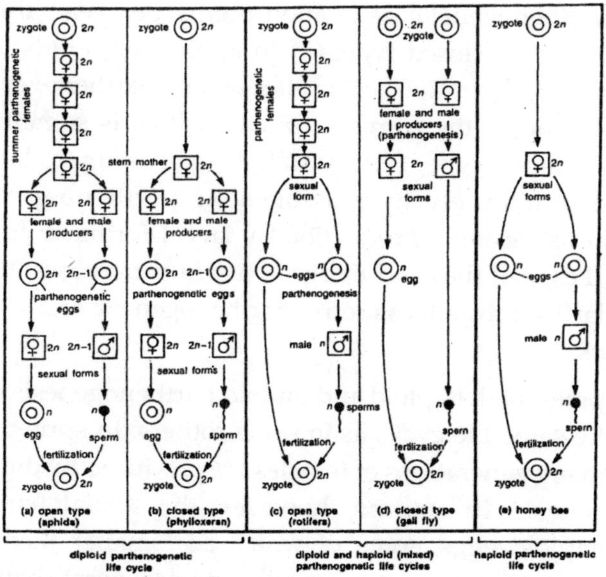

Different kinds of parthenogenetic life cycle in animal.

Obligate Diploid Parthenogenesis: Populations originating through obligate parthenogenesis consist of only females. Males, whenever present are generally non-functional. In this type of parthenogenesis, meiosis is either lacking (apomictic or ameiotic thelytoky) or the meiosis may be followed by a compensating process restoring the diploid chromosome number (automictic or meiotic thelytoky). In automictic thelytoky, the diploid chromosome number is restored either by fusion of the ovum with a polar body or by the fusion of the two cleavage nuclei. This provides a mechanism to generate genetic variability despite parthenogenesis.

Cyclical Parthenogenesis: Sometimes partheno-genesis alternates with sexual reproduction in a cycle and is then described as cyclical. Several variations occur in this alternation of sexual and parthenogenetic generations (Fig.). Some of these variations include the following: (i) In gall flies (Cynipidae, Hymenoptera), an alternation between one sexual generation and one parthenogenetic generation occurs per year; this is often described as closed type, (ii) In aphids; daphnids, and rotifers, asexual generation occurs after several parthenogenetic generations during the summer of a year; this is sometimes described as open type, (iii) In *Miaster* (gall midge),, larvae reproduce indefinitely by paedogenetic partheno-genesis (paedogenesis means reproduction by larval forms as found in liver flukes, gall flies and midges), (iv) In some cases, there is no regularity in the alternation of parthenogenetic and sexual generations.

Sometimes, both haploid and diploid parthenogenesis may occur in the same life cycle, as in some rotifers. In spring and summer, many generations of females are produced by diploid parthenogenesis. In autumn, however, the sexual females produce haploid eggs, some of which are smaller than the others and develop parthenogenetically into degenerate haploid males, that produce spermatozoa. The larger eggs are fertilized and produce zygotes with thick shells to overcome the unfavourable conditions. In the following spring, these diploids develop into females parthenogenetically.

Haploid Parthenogenesis (arrhenotoky): Haploid parthenogenesis involves production of haploid ova which develop into haploid embryos without fertilization. In some species, haploid parthenogenesis also works as a mechanism of sex determination. For instance, in Hymenoptera (bees, wasps, ants), Coleoptera (few species of beetles). Coccoidea (scale insects), Aleurodoidae (white flies), Hemiptera (some of the bugs), and Arachnida (mite), unfertilised eggs develop into males, and fertilised eggs develop into females.

Since, both parthenogenetic haploids and sexual diploids exist in these animals, the condition is also described as haplodiploidy or arrhenotoky. Normal meiosis can not occur in haploid males of these animals.

They produce sperms by skipping the first meiotic division and forming two sperm cells through second meiosis. In these animals (as demonstrated in *Habrobracon)*, diploid males could also be produced in the laboratory, from homozygous diploid eggs, so that the males can be either homozygous diploids or hemizygous haploids and the females are heterozygous diploids.

'In honey bees *(Apis)*, there are three types of individuals: (i) the diploid fertile female queen (develops from fertlized egg, where the larvae are fed on special food called 'royal jelly'), (ii) the diploid sterile female workers (develop from fertilized eggs), and (iii) the fertile haploid males called drones (develop parthenogenetically, from haploid unfertilised eggs without fertilization).

Reproduction in Plant Systems: In lower plant species (algae, fungi, bryophytes), the gametophyte is the dominant free living generation. However, the gametophytes of angiosperms (which will be discussed in this section) are smaller and less complex than the corresponding sporophytes. These gametophytes are formed within the specialised organs of the flower. The male gametophyte develops within the anther, while the female gametophyte develops within the ovule. Sexual reproduction requires that the sperm nuclei developed in the male gametophyte (pollen) are delivered to the embryo sac, where fertilization occurs and the new diploid sporophyte is formed. A wealth of information about the sexual reproduction in these higher plants (angiosperms) has been obtained using genetic and molecular analyses of pollen development, embryo sac development, pollen-stigma/style interactions.

Anther vs. Pollen

Male reproductive processes occur in the anther, which is a part of stamen, that consists of a filament and an anther. The filament is a tube, which anchors the stamen to the flower and serves as a conduit for water and nutrients. Anthers, on the other hand, contain reproductive and nonreproductive tissues, that are responsible for producing and releasing pollen grains, each of them containing a male gametophyte.

The development of male gametophyte may be completed before or even after the pollen grains are released from the anther. In either case, the pollen grain with male gametophyte loses contact with anther walls; before it brings about pollination and fertilization.

Anther Development: Anther development can be divided into two phases (Fig). During phase 1, anther develops and differentiates, and microspore mother cells undergo meiosis, so that at the end of phase 1, anther contains all its specialised cells and tissues including tetrads of microspores that are present within the pollen sacs.

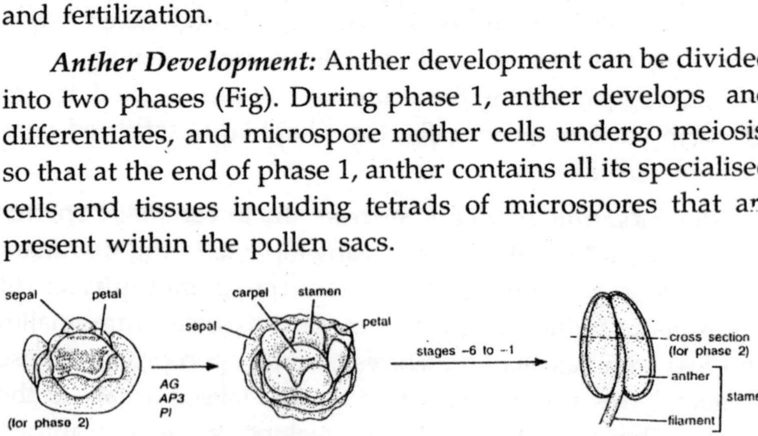

(a) phase 1 involving (i) cell specification, (ii) tissue differentiation and (iii) meiosis and spore formation

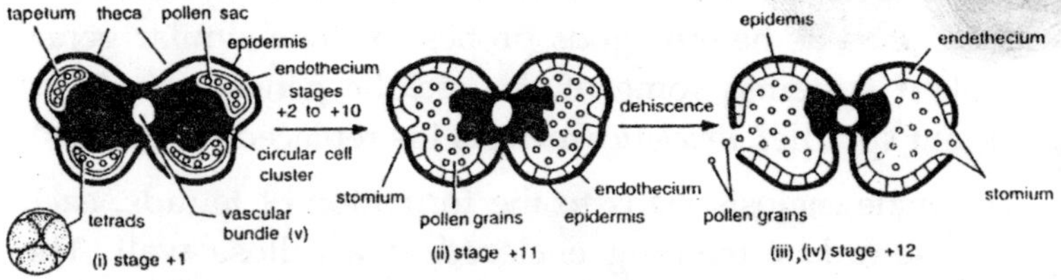

(b) phase 2 involving (i) pollen grain and sperm cell defferentiation; (ii) anther enlargement and filament extension, (iii) tissue degeneration and (iv) dehiscence and pollen release.

Different stages of anther development involving two phases (redrawn form 'The plant Cell', October 1993).

During phase 2, pollen grains differentiate and mature, anther enlarges in size, filament elongates, tissues inside the anther degenerate and the anther undergoes dehiscence releasing the pollen grains. Cellular processes leading to switch from phase 1 to phase 2 are not fully understood, but some information has become available in the recent past.

Stamen primorida are initiated as a whorl of small bumps at specific locations on the surface of floral meristem. Initiation of these primordia does not depend upon the presence of sepal or petal primorida. Several homeotic genes involved in the process include *APETALA3 (AP3), PISTILLATA (PI)* and AGAMOUS (AG) in *Arabidopsis*, their counterparts in snapdragon being *DEFICIENS (DEF), GLOBOSA (GLO)* and *PLENA (PLE)*. Related homeotic genes are also known in tobacco, petunia, tomato and corn. Mutations in any of these genes result in loss of stamen primordia and their conversion into primordia for another floral whorl. Most of these genes encode transcription factors. Mitochondrial genome has also been shown to be involved in anther development.

Microsporogenesis and Development of Male Gametophyte : Microsporogenesis starts with a diploid sporophytic cell, which divides to form (i) the tapetal initial and (ii) the sporogenous initial (pollen mother cell). The sporogenous cell divides by a meiotic division having several events controlled by independent genes. These events include entry into meiosis, synapsis, recombination, spindle formation, etc. The genes for these events have been cloned from some animal systems and could be used as heterologous probes to clone similar genes from plant systems. Some of the meiotic genes include *dv* (divergent spindle), *ameiotic* (meiosis I is replaced by mitosis).

The male meiosis leads to the formation of tetrads, each of these tetrads remaining enclosed in a callose wall. The callase produced from the tapetum breaks the callose wall releasing the microspores described as pollen grains. The pollen wall formation starts soon after meiosis and consists of exine made up of sporopo Uenin and intine made up of pectocellulose. The exine also has "patterns of spines, netlike ridges or other projections. The pollen wall sculpturing is determined during meiosis and callose wall plays a role in this pattern formation. The pollen also has pores, where pollen tube grows. These pores may have correlation with the meiotic spindle poles and exine deposition is reduced or absent at these pores.

Each microspore divides by an asymmetric mitotic division forming a larger vegetative cell and a smaller generative cell. In -70% of plant families, the pollen grains are released from the anther at this 2-celled stage and the second mitotic division producing two sperm cells from a generative cell occurs when the pollen tube grows (Fig.). But in families like Cruciferae and Gramineae, this second mitotic division also occurs before the pollen is released from the anther. The sperm cells together with the vegetative nucleus constitute what is sometimes described as 'male germ unit' or MGU. The two sperm cells are not always similar. One is associated with the vegetative nucleus and the other lies behind it. Sperm dimorphism has also been observed in some cases. Both cytoplasmic heterospermy and nuclear heterospermy have been observed. Nuclear heterospermy is generally due to presence or absence of B chromosomes and has been reported in maize only.

The generative cell, and the resulting sperm cells contain few mitochondria, sparse ER, condensed chromatin and fewer nuclear pores in their nuclei.

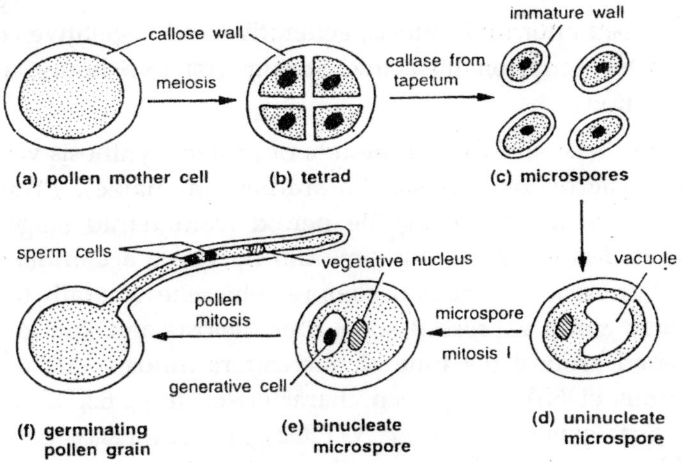

Microsporgenesis and the development of a male gemetophyte in a typical Angiosperm.

This suggests that these nuclei are transcriptionally less active than the vegetative cell nucleus. There is also evidence of association between vegetative nucleus and the generative/ sperm cells. In some cases, it has been shown that there are more nuclear pores on the surface of the vegetative nucleus which is appressed to the generative cell implying communication between the two. Evidence is also available for gene expression specific to vegetative nucleus. It is also speculated that cell cycle genes (*e.g.*, cyclin genes) must be specifically expressed in the generative cell, but not in the vegetative cell. It has also been shown that the generative cell can be isolated and cultured so that it can undergo mitosis without any association with vegetative cell. At the surface of the generative cell or sperm cells are also expressed epitopes which may help in sperm-egg cell recognition.

Mature pollen contains proteins synthesised during maturation, and the mRNAs synthesised earlier. These mRNAs seem to be under translational control (compare with animal systems, where maternal mRNAs are preferentially translated), but no detailed studies about their localisation within the cell and preferential translation have been conducted. When pollen are released after first mitosis, generative and vegetative cells remain transcriptionally active during first two hours after germination.

It has been shown that the rate of protein synthesis varies during microsporogenesis (as studied in maize). Protein synthesis is active during the period from tetrad stage to vacuolated microspore; it is slow during starch accumulation period and is active again just before dehiscene. Actually there are early genes expressed soon after meiosis and late genes expressed around the time of microspore mitosis. Although numerous cDNAs have been characterised (*e.g., E2, 13, Bp4, Bp10, Bcp1* genes in *Brsssica; NTP303* gene in tobacco *LAT51, LAT52, LAT56, LAT59* genes of tomato), but more work is needed to isolate specific genes that are expressed for specific short intervals during microsporogenesis.

Genes for cytcskeleton organisation have also been isolated. Actin filaments appear around the plasma membrane oriented with cellulose fibrils of the intine and also around the generative and vegetative nuclei. It has also been shown that heat shock response is expressed in immature pollen, but not in the mature pollen. It is speculated that the transcription factors specific to heat shock genes may be absent in mature pollen. In tomato, heat shock specific transcription factors have actually been isolated. Further study of these transcription factors will throw light on the mechanism of the heat shock response in immature pollen and the absence of such a response in mature pollen.

Ovule vs. Embryo Sac

In comparison to male gametophyte, relatively less is known about the regulation of female gametophyte development. The ovule contains the megagmetophyte and itself develops into the seed. The differentiation of megasporocyte (megaspore mother cell), production of functional megaspore (megasporogenesis), formation of embryo sac (megagametogenesis) and embryogenesis all occur within the ovule. Unlike pollen, which is released and loses contact with anther wall, embryo sacs maintain physical contact with the sporophyte (ovule) throughout their development. This provides an opportunity to examine interactions between cells, tissues and genomes.

Ovule Development: The ovule develops as a specialised structure from the placenta of the ovary wall. It consists of nucellus, integument(s) and the funiculus. The nucellus (derived from apical portion of the ovule primordium) functions as megasporangium, producing the megasporocyte which undergoes meiosis to form megaspores. After ovule initiation, a single subdermal nucellar cell enlarges and is seen to have a prominent nucleus.

This cell represents archesporium, although multicellular archesporium containing several archesporial cells are also known in soyabean and *Brassica campestris*. The single cell representing the archesporium may directly function as megasporocyte or may undergo -a division to form a megasporocyte and a somatic cell. When multicellular archesporium is present, one archesporial cell functions as the megaspore mother cell.

In ~65% of species examined, most of the nucellus degenerates before the embryo sac reaches maturity, thus bringing the embryo sac in direct contact of the integument. In such cases, the innermost layer of integument differentiates into endothelium, which resembles tapetum in the anther, and performs a similar nutritional function. In the remaining ~35% species, the nucellus does not degenerate, no endothelium is differentiated and the embryo sac receives nutrients directly from the nucellus. The funiculus connects the ovule with ovary wall, and the micropyle is located at the points where integuments terminate and pollen tube enters the ovule. This organisation provides ovular polarity in the development of embryo sac.

Embryo sac Development (Megasporogenesis and Megagametogenesis): Embryo sac development consists of megasporogenesis and megagametogenesis. The megasporogenesis involves meiosis giving four nuclei for four megaspores. Subsequent mitotic divisions, nuclear migration and cytokinesis, collectively described as megagametogenesis, produce the embryo sac, which exhibits considerable diversity among species (Fig.).

Approximately 70% of the species examined including *Aqibidopsis* and maize possess *Polygonum* type of embryo sac, which develops from the functional megaspore located at the chalazal end of the ovule (from a linear tetrad three micropylar megaspores degenerate).

The functional megaspore undergoes three successive mitotic divisions to produce eight nuclei. This functional megaspore is selected with the help of callose (a (β -1,3-glucan), because the callose walls become thinner or absent in the functional megaspore and are thick and persistent in the degenerating megaspores.

The absence of callose allows flow of nutrients thus facilitating this megaspore to become functional. The eight nucleate *Polygonum* type of embryo sac is organised into 3 antipodals at one pole, 2 synergids and one egg cell at the other pole and two polar nuclei at the centre (Fig.).

Cytological and cytochemical studies have also been undertaken to localise the presence of proteins, starch, lipids and nucleic acids in the different cells of the embryo sac. These studies allowed the assessment of the physiological state of the embryo sac and the rates of metabolic activity of different cells of the embryo sac.

The presence of numerous ribosomes and mitochondria in the synergids, central cells and the antipodals suggest a high rate of metabolic activity in these cells. On the other hand, the egg cell is relatively quiescent as evident from the presence of fewer ribosomes, plastids and other organelles in this cell. However, very little information is available about the temporal and spatial patterns of gene expression in the embryo sac. The molecular and genetic studies are just beginning, which will answer many questions in the future.

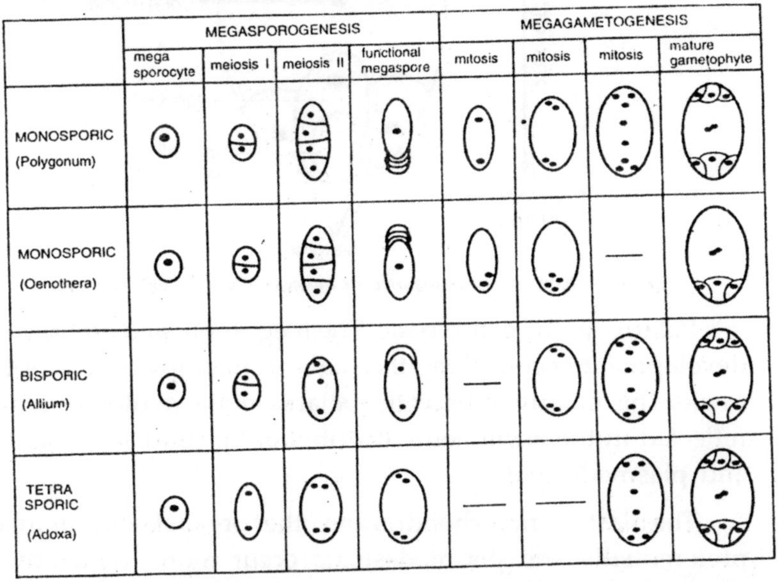

Organisation of a monosporic Polygonum type of embryo sac development, representative genera are indicated in parantheses below the types in the first column.

The mature embryo sacs of different species differ, depending upon whether one, two or four megaspore nuclei contribute to their formation. However, the functional organisation of cells at the micropylar end of the embryo sac is remarkably similar showing one egg, two synergids and a central cell. The only exceptions are:

(i) peperomia type, which forms only one synergid and

(ii) plumbago and plumbagella types, which form no synergids.

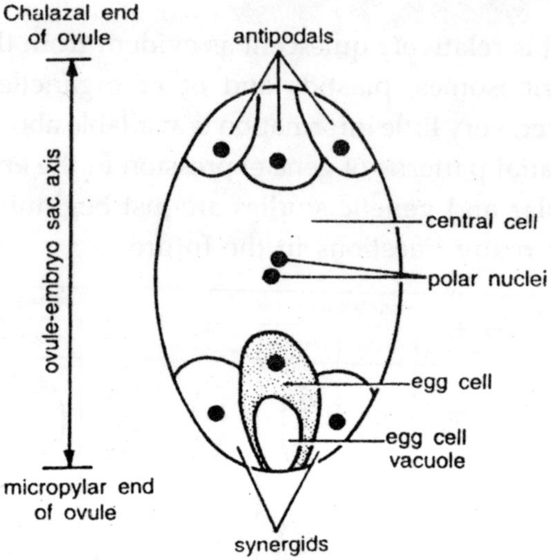

Organisation of a monosporic Polygonum type of embryo sac.

Polarity in the embryo sac. The megaspore and embryo sac development occurs along the chalazal-micropylar axis of the ovule. This polarity reflects the polarity of the ovule and is also reflected in the asymmetric distribution of cellular organelles and plasmodesmata.

The plastids, mitochondria and other organelles accumulate preferentially and plasmodesmata occur more frequently at the chalazal end of megaspore mother cell (megasporocyte), so that most of the organelles are inherited by the chalazal most cell after the first meiotic division. After meiosis, plastids are preferentially distributed at the micropylar end of the functional megaspore and plasmodesmata are usually observed only between the functional megaspore and the nucellus. The functional megaspore thus inherits a richer cytoplasm and preferentially receives nutrients from the maternal cytoplasm. The cytoskeleton also plays a role in the distribution of cytoplasmic contents during megasporogenesis and megagametogenesis.

In the embryo sac, synergids often have elaborate wall

projections called filiform apparatus that extends into the nucellus and provide a mechanism for nutrient flow from the ovule to the embryo sac. Wall projections also extend from the antipodal cells into the chalazal nucellus. This represents another site for metabolite flow from the nucellus to the embryo sac. Differences in the nutritional status at the two ends of the embryo sac actually influences the development and positioning of the egg and synergids.

In the mature embryo sac, the most notable expression of polarity is found in the egg cell. The micropylar portion of egg cell is occupied by a vacuole. The nucleus, cytoplasm and most of the organelles are found at the chalazal end.

Cellularisation of Embryo Sac: Cellularisation of embryo sac, which follows meiotic division, is the most poorly understood part of megagametophyte development. It may involve formation of two, three or four cell plates according to three different models. All these models propose formation of one cell plate between two synergids and the other between the egg apparatus and the central cell.

The egg cell may be separated from the synergids by a common cell wall or by two separate cell walls. After the cell wall formation, the egg and synergids are poorly differentiated from each other. Each cell is small and wedge shaped with a flattened chalazal wall. Each of these cells expands towards the chalaza, inflating into a rounded cell with different placements, the egg cell towards the chalazal end, and the synergids towards the micropylar end of the egg apparatus.

The cell walls between egg cell and synergids eventually become discontinuous with bead-like structures separated by segments of closely appressed plasma membranes. At the micropylar end of the synergids, cell wall ingrowths are formed, thus giving rise to a distinctive filiform apparatus (FA), which identifies the synergids. The egg apparatus together with the central nucleus is described as the female germ unit (FGU), which is required to affect double fertilization. The FGU extends the concept of egg apparatus to include in it the egg apparatus and the central cell. The components of FGU attract and receive the pollen tube, cause the sperm cells to be discharged and transported in the female gametophyte. It also helps in the fusion of one sperm with the egg cell and the other with the central cell.

The normal intact FGU is characterised by the presence of (i) narrow micropylar entries (checking entry of supernumerary pollen tubes which may cause polyspermy) ; (ii) cytoskeletal elements within and between cells (which guide the migration of male nuclei) ; (iii) poorly developed cell walls (at the point of entry of sperms) in egg cell and central cell and (iv) the proximity of egg and polar nuclei at the time of fusion. Like the FGU, the male reproductive unit in the male gametophyte is called 'male germ unit' (MGU) which consists of the vegetative nucleus and the sperm cells.

Egg Cell: The egg cell, is similar to synergids in cell shape. It is so placed, that it is not penetrated by the pollen tube. The pollen tube actually pushes the synergids, ruptures one of them and releases the sperms there, from where they are transferred into the egg and the central cell. The cell wall of egg cell at its chalazal end is incomplete over one half to two third of the cell to facilitate contact with synergids and central cell.

Between the egg cell and the central cell there is present high level of actin. Two actin 'coronas' are observed, one above the chalazal end of the egg and the other over the synergids. Mature egg cell has a large and regular nucleus (larger in size than those of synergids) located at its chalazal end and a centrally located vacuole that is surrounded by a large number of smaller vacuoles. The egg nucleus also has a large nucleolus with high potential for the production of ribosomes. Although most egg cells are poor in Golgi apparatus, they show variation in the distribution and abundance of plastids (varying from 8 to 730 in a egg cell), micothondria (ranging from. 1000 to 40,000 per egg cell) and ER.

Receipt of the Pollen Tube, Release of Sperms and Double Fertilization: The synergids which receive the pollen tube and the sperms, work as a source of chemical signal that diverts the pollen tube to enter the micropyle, penetrate one synergid and release its gametes there. Myosin is present in the pollen tube on the surface of the organelles and on the generative/ sperm cells. The actin bundles in the cytoplasm of pollen tube interact with myosin on the surface of the organelles. This propels the male cells through the tube and maintains association of male cells with the vegetative nucleus.

The pollen tube enters the degenerated synergid and the released male gametes move into the chalazal end of the synergid. The interaction between 'myosin' on the surface of male gametes and 'actin coronas' help in movement of sperm cells. The plasma membranes of sperm cells fuse with those of target female cell (egg cell or central cell). For this fusion, either specific fusogenic receptors or divalent cations (Ca^{++}) are needed. The sperm nuclei are thus transferred one each into the egg cell and the central cell, which is followed by migration and alignment of these nuclei to bring about nuclear fusion. The outer membrane of the nuclei fuse first, followed by the fusion of inner membranes. The fusion of nucleoplasms, then completes the fusion process.

The sperm cells may exhibit cytoplasmic or nuclear heterospermy. This may lead to preferential fertilization. In *Plumbago,* the sperm associated with vegetative nucleus is designated as *Svn,* which contains no plastids, but contains 200 mitochondria and the other is designated as *Sua* (unassociated), which contains 24 plastids and 50 mitochondria. The plastid rich *Sua* fuses with egg (94% of the times) and selectively transmits male plastids into the zygote. However, the ratio of male and female mitochondria (1:1000), however, remains the same in fertilized egg and the central cell, due to similar differences in mitochondria in the two sperm cells and those between unfertilised egg and the central cell. In maize, when there is nuclear heterospermy, sperm containing B chromosome preferentially fuses with the egg cell, although presence of too many B-chromosomes or the presence of an A-B translocation in the maternal genotype may negate this effect. The fertilization may also fail due to the presence of a specific gene (*'hap'* in barley) in the female genotype. Fertilization in plants, as in animals, is accompanied by dramatic changes in Ca^{++} concentration. Ca^{++} ions in high concentration are released during the degeneration of the synergid and the collapse of vacuole. This high concentration of Ca^{++} in degenerated synergids influences the environment for fusion of gametes and thus affects fertilization and post-fertilization events.

Genetic and Molecular Analysis of Ovule and Embryo Sac Development: Mutations affecting development of the ovule and embryo sac have been identified by screening plants with reduced fertility. They can be expressed either in the parent sporophyte affecting all embryo sacs in a plant or in an ovule, or in the gametophyte (embryo sac) itself. Therefore, they can be classified into sporophytic and gametophytic mutants.

Sporophytic Mutants: Some of the representative female-sterile mutants affecting development of ovule/embryo sacs have been detected in *Arabidopsis* and include the following : (i) short integument-1 or *sin-1,* where meiosis occurs, but normal tetrads and embryo sacs are not formed; (ii) ovule mutant-3 *(ovm-3)* lack both integuments, and the products of meiosis, degenerate; (iii) ovule mutant-2 *(ovm-2),* where both integuments are present, but space normally occupied by embryo sac is filled with nucellar cells, and (iv) *bel-1,* which lacks inner integument, so that a functional embryo sac is not produced. Thus *sinl* and *ovm3* exhibit abnormal Tegasporogenesis while *bell* and *ovm2* exhibit aborted megagametogenesis. Additional mutations will be studied in future, which will define the interactions between the ovule and the embryo sac.

Sporophytic mutants have also been detected in which meiosis is disrupted. In maize meiotic mutants *(mei)* have been shown to affect several aspects of meiosis including the following: (i) initiation of meiosis, (ii) control of meiotic divisions; (iii) pairing of homologous chromosomes and (iv) mitotic divisions within the gametophyte. Defects in meiosis may also lead to the formation of diploid apomictic embryo sacs. For instance dyad mutant in *Datura* blocks meiosis II, creating a dyad of unreduced megaspores giving diploid embryo sacs.

Gametophytic Mutants: This class of mutants depends on the haploid genotype of the embryo sac and includes the following: (i) indeterminate gametophyte *(ig)* in maize, where the multiple functional egg cells and embryos are produced and develop into haploids without fertilization;(ii) gametophytic expression *(Gf)* in *Arabidopsis,* where the genes linked to *Gf* have reduced transmission through the female gametophyte, suggesting that mutant gametophytes are less viable than the wild type. (Reduced transmission could also be due to linkage of *Gf* with a structural change in chromosome). These and other gametophytic mutants along with sporophytic mutants will greatly help in defining the pathways of ovule and embryo sac development.

Molecular Analysis: Following are some examples, where molecular aspects of ovule and embryo sac development were examined. These studies will certainly be expanded in future: (i) pistil specific mRNA (pMON 9608) was located in the integuments of tomato ovules by in-situ hybridisation; (ii) mRNA for *AGAMOUS (AG)* and *APETALA3* in *Arabidopsis* encoding transcription factors were located in endothelium and integuments respectively; (iii) AC-like genes *AGL1* and *AGL2* are expressed in the ovules of *Arabidopsis.* Only future studies will demonstrate the roles of these genes/mRNAs in ovule and embryo sac development.

Apomixis: In the past, the term apomixis (apo=without; mixis=fusion of gametes), as against amphimixis (meaning fusion of two types of gametes), has been used to describe all kinds of asexual reproduction including vegetative propagation. In recent years, however, apomixis is being used in a more restricted sense, to include only those processes of asexual reproduction, which lead to the formation of fertile botanic seed without any fusion of male and female gametes.

The term agamospermy was earlier used to describe these processes, so that apomixis in the past included both agamospermy and vegetative propagation. The development of embryos in apomixis also differs from that of the embryos produced due to somatic embryogenesis, which involves a callus phase and where the patterns of embryo formation is very different than that in sexual or apomictic embryos developing in the ovule.

In view of the above, if apomixis can be artificially induced in crop plants, this can be of immense use in perpetuating an elite genotype, and in maintaining characteristics like heterosis. The apomictic'embryos are thus solely derived from the maternal tissue within the ovule, and therefore, barring differences due to mutations, have a genetic constitution similar to that of the female parent. Due to its relevance to heterosis breeding, apomixis research in crop plants attracted renewed emphasis in recent years.

Apomixis has been reported in at least 300 plant species belonging to 35 families, more prominent of these families being Graminase (Poaceae), Compositae (Asteraceae) and Rosaceae. However, apomixis is not common in agriculturally important plant species except in apple and *Citrus*. Further, the attempts to transfer or induce apomixis in agricultural crops' have so far been unsuccessful, except some success achieved in pearl millet.

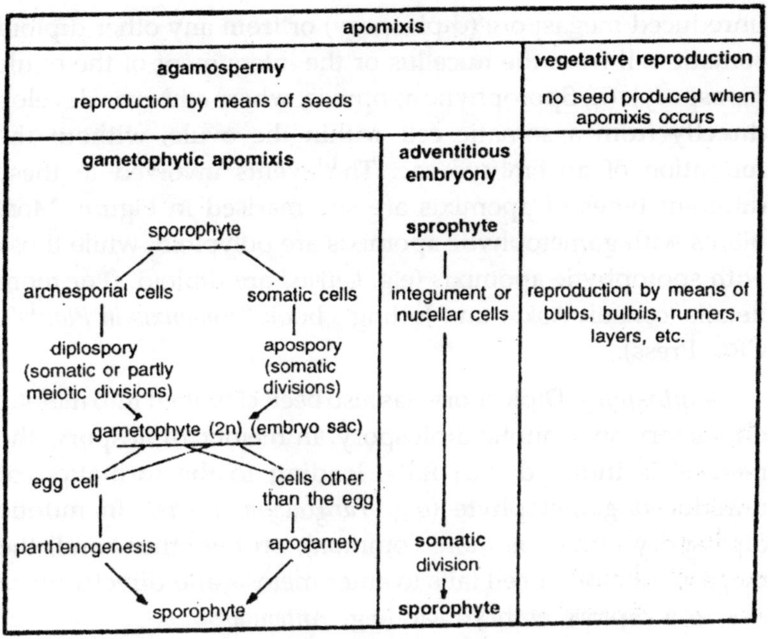

A classification of different types of apomisis in flowering plants.

Three steps in apomixis (failure of meiosis, failure of fertilization and parthenogenesis). The development of seed through apomixis involves the following steps: (i) failure of meiosis or avoiding meiosis, leading to the development of unreduced gametophyte (or direct development of embryo without any gametophytic stage); (ii) failure of fertilization of unreduced female gamete; and (iii) parthenogenetic development of the embryo from unfertilised and unreduced eggs. As we know, occurrence of any one of these three events in sexual species will lead to failure of the development of viable seed. But in apomicts, these aberrant events are successfully completed to produce viable seed that are maternal in their genetic constitution.

Two Major Types of Apomixis: Apomixis may be of the following two types: (i) Gametophytic apomixis, where an embryo sac (female gametophyte) is produced, either from the unreduced megaspore (diplospory) or from any other diploid somatic cell from the nucellus or the integument of the ovule (apospory). (ii) Sporophytic apomixis, where embryos develop directly from a somatic cell within the ovule, without the formation of an embryo sac. The events involved in these different types of apomixis are summarised in Figure. Most plants with gametophytic apomixis are polyploid, while those with sporophytic apomixis (e.g. *Citrus)* are diploid. (For more details, consult Asker and Jerling's book *"Apomixis in Plants"*, CRC Press).

Diplospory: Diplospory has also been classified into meiotic diplospory and mitotic diplospory. In meiotic diplospory, the meiosis is initiated, but fails, leading to the formation of unreduced gametophyte (e.g. *Taraxacum, Ixeris).* In mitotic diplospory (which is more common), on the other hand, the megaspore mother cell fails to enter meiosis and directly gives rise to a diploid embryo sac (e.g. *Antennaria).*

Apospory: Aposporic embryo sacs develop from additional cells that differentiate from the nucellus, and do not involve the archesporial cell or megaspore mother cell. These cells are called aposporic initials and give rise to unreduced aposporic embryo sacs (which are often more than one in an ovule), by mitotic divisions. These aposporic sacs can coexist with sexual embryo sacs. (In diplospory, diplosporous unreduced embryo sacs can not co-exist with sexual reduced embryo sacs). The aposporous initials generally develop in a zone adjacent to the megaspore mother cell (mmc). This suggests that either the signal that specifies mmc has been expanded or a restriction imposed, preventing differentiation of more than one megaspore mother cells. The aposporic embryo sacs often resemble their sexual counterparts in the number of nuclei and their arrangement. However, in Gramineae, aposporic embryo sacs are often unipolar and have only four nuclei (or sometimes only two nuclei) at one pole, in contrast to the sexual sacs, which are typical bipolar *Polygonum* type with proliferating antipodals on one pole and the egg apparatus on the other pole.

Parthenogenesis and Apogamety (pseudogamy vs autonomy): Both in diplosporous and aposporous apomictic embryo sacs, the nuclei are diploid. In these embryo sacs, no fertilization occurs, and the embryo develops directly either from the egg (parthenogenesis) or from any other cell of the embryo sac (apogamety).

The embryo development is accompanied with endosperm development from the central cell. The endosperm development may be autonomous (no pollination is necessary) as in most of the diplosporous apomicts (particularly the members of Compositae) and in some rare aposporous apomicts (*e.g. Hieracium* species). In these cases, embryo development generally starts before anthesis (dehiscence of anthers). Alternatively, the endosperm development may be pseudogamous (pollination is necessary and selective fusion takes place between an unreduced polar nucleus and a sperm nucleus) as in most of the aposporous apomicts and in some diplosporous grasses (*e.g. Elymus, Poa, Eragrostis* and *Tripsacum).*

When the pollination takes place in pseudogamous apomicts, the pollen tube enters into only one of the several embryo sacs available. This favoured embryo sac, generally is the one, which is located at the most favourable position, *i.e.* closest to the micropylar end. This leads to fusion of one sperm nucleus with the central cell involving two polar nuclei. Only rarely, the unreduced egg cell is also fertilized leading to increase in ploidy level in the progeny (*e.g. Poa).* The mechanism that prevents fertilization is unknown, but this lack of fertilization of the egg is certainly not coupled with the production of unreduced embryo sacs.

Adventive Embryony: Adventitious embryos may develop either from the nucellar cells or from the cells of the integument. Nucellar embryony is more common and is found in *Citrus,* the model system for this type of embryo development. In *Citrus,* sexual and apomictic development of embryos occur concurrently even within the same ovule. The necellar cells destined to develop directly into the embryos are characterised by large nuclei and dense cytoplasm. As the initials differentiate, a callose wall forms within the original primary cell wall. In some *Citrus* cultivars, as many as 50 such initials may differentiate in a single ovule. However, only the initial cells located in the micropylar region divide and form embryos. The fertilized embryo sac appears to have inhibitory influence on nucellar embryogenesis in the chalazal region. Even in sexual embryo sac, embryos develop at the micropylar end, and are inhibited in the chalazal region. The *Citrus* seeds are generally polyembryonic having embryos derived both from sexual embryo sacs and those developed due to adventive embryony.

Genetics of Apomixis: Genetics of apomixis has been worked out in several cases through crosses between sexual forms and apomicts (used as male parent). Following are some conclusions: (i) In *Citrus,* nucellar embryony is controlled by a single dominant gene, (ii) In *Pennisetum, Panicum,* and *Ranunculus* apospory is controlled by a single dominant gene, (iii) In some other cases (*Dichanthium-Bothriochloa* complex), more than one gene are suggested to control apomixis. According to an earlier hypothesis there are three genes, one controlling meiosis and development of gametophyte, the other controlling lack of fertilization and the third controlling, development of egg into embryo. In any case, apomixis does not seem to be controlled by many genes, although the effects are profound.

Models for the gene expression controlling apomixis have also been proposed. Popular models assume that the proteins needed for sexual pathway get altered in apomicts and that perhaps no novel, proteins are needed for apomixis. According to Peacock (1992), apomictic gene (embryo sac inducer gene = *Esi)* produces a transcriptional activator needed for normal development. Precocious expression of this gene in mmc or its expression in cells (nucellar cells), where it is not supposed to be expressed, may lead to diplospory/apospory. There may be additional genes for autogamy/pseudogamy and for parthenogenesis. No gene for apomictic reproduction has been isolated so far and, therefore, the identity of gene products and their functions remain unknown. However, tagging of a gene for apomixis has been possible in *Pennisetum*. Apospory in the genus *Pennisetum*, was also successfully transferred from *P. squamulatum* to sexual species, the cultivated pearl-millet. The resultant apomictic line in BC3 had a single supernumerary chromosome containing gene for apomixis from *P. squamulatum*. RFLP molecular markers (RFLP=restriction fragment length polymorphism; linked to apospory, were also identified in this BC_3 population. Similar studies were also conducted in *Potentilla* and *Rubus* using DNA fingerprinting.

Molecular Mechanisms for Sexual and Apomictic Developmental Pathways: Unfortunately, nothing is known so far, about the similarities and differences between genes expressed during apomictic and sexual developmental pathways. One may, however, speculate the following two mechanisms: (i) There may be a substrate product relationship, in which an early event produces a component, that is essential for a subsequent event, thus suggesting the dependence of a subsequent event on the completion of the previous event. (ii) There may be feedback controls, which keep the early event under surveillance, so that without the completion of this event, no signal can be sent to an active controlling system or checkpoint. Mutations in the feedback control may thus uncouple any two sequential events (e.g. fertilization and development of embryo). In apomixis, only endosperm development may be dependent on fertilization (as in pseudogamy), but embryo sac formation and embryo formation do not depend on meiosis and/or fertilization. It is believed that a feedback control system that operates in sexual reproduction is disrupted in apomicts. This is perhaps achieved by presentation of a signal to the checkpoint that commits a fraud in telling the checkpoint that the event is complete, even when it is not completed. At the cellular level, an important difference in the sexual and apomictic developmental pathways involves formation of callose walls.

The observations summarised in Table suggest that there are differences in callose cell walls between sexual and apomictic pathways, indicating that callose wall may be necessary for meiosis to take place and its absence may be required for the development of the gametophyte from its initials (megaspore or aposporic initial). More studies at the molecular level may be needed to dissect out precisely the factors at the cellular level, which are responsible for apomictic seed formation.

Differences between Sexual and Apomictic Pathways for Callose wall Formation and for the Presence/absence of some Specific Proteins.

Sexual Pathway	*Apomictic Pathway*
A callose wall is formed around mine before meiosis;	No callose wall around mine in diplosporous apomicts, and incomplete callose wall around mmc in aposporous apomicts;
Chalazal functional megaspore lacks callose wall, but other three megaspores have callose walls	Aposporous embryo sac initials lack callose walls
Callose wall around developing sexual embryos	Cellose wall around developing aposporic embryos
A protein (MAC207-reactive epitope) present in all somatic tissues is absent in the nuceliar cells	Not studied in apomicts
The nucellar cells lacking the above protein contain another arabinogalactan protein (JIMB-reactive epitope), which is also found on the surface of sperm cells, egg cell and the synergids, but absent from vegetative cell in the pollen, antipodals and the central cells	Not studied in apomicts

10

Bacteria and Tissues

For long time, bacteria and viruses were believed to reproduce through purely asexual methods, so that these organisms did not make suitable material for genetic studies. In the year 1946, two American scientists, J. Lederberg and E.L. Tatum demonstrated sexuality in bacteria for the first time, and this opened a new area of research. For this and other contributions, Lederberg and Tatum shared with G.W. Beadle the Nobel Prize in medicine, for the year 1958.

Once sexuality in bacteria was established, short generation time and several other facilities which these organisms provided, made them very suitable materials for genetic studies. As a result of work on these organisms great advances have been made in the field of cell biology, molecular biology and genetics in the second half of 20th century. A brief account of cell biology and basic genetics of these organisms will be presented in this chapter.

Three Methods for Transfer of Genetic Material: Sexuality and recombination in bacteria will involve transfer of genetic material from one bacterial cell to another. Following three methods for such a transfer are known and are illustrated in Figure. (i) *Transformation*: In this case, genetic material is released from one strain and a part may be acquired from another strain, which thus gets transformed without coming in contact with the other strain (Fig.A), (ii) *Transduction*: In this phenomenon, a virus when released from a host bacterial strain may carry with it a part of genetic material of the host strain and may transfer it to another strain later infected by this virus (Fig. B), (iii) *Conjugation:* In this case, genetic material is transferred through a conjugation tube, when two strains come in contact (Fig.C).

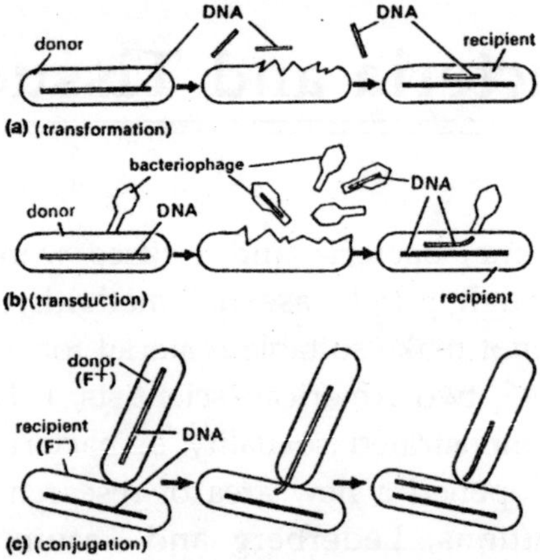

Three different methods for transfer of genetic material from one bacterial strain to another bacterial strain.

Sexual Combination in Bacteria

Culture Media and Mutant Strains: Most of the important work on genetics of bacteria was at least initially done on colon bacillus *(Escherichia coli = E. coli)*. These bacteria can be grown in petri-dishes or in culture tubes on a simple culture medium consisting of glucose, ammonium salts and a few additional substances needed in traces. From these simple substances, other complicated substances like vitamins and amino acids can be manufactured by the bacteria themselves. The strains of bacteria which can grow on this simplest medium, are called prototrophs. However, certain mutant strain may be incapable of manufacturing a particular substance, so that this specific substance will have to be added to the simplest (minimal) medium for the growth of the mutant strain.

Such a mutant strain is called an auxotroph. Other kinds of mutants may also be available. For instance a strain may be a mutant for its capacity to resist infection by a virus or it may be resistant to an antibiotic like streptomycin. These resistant strains are though mutants, can still grow on minimal medium and will therefore be called prototrophs and not auxotrophs.

Bacteria can be grown either in liquid medium or on the surface of medium which is made solid by means of agar (a gelatin like substance). In liquid medium, cells will always remain scattered, but on a solid medium, the products of cell division will remain together to form a colony, so that ultimately each colony will represent descendants of a single cell (Fig.). Availability of these culture techniques enable detection of a few prototrophs among millions of cells. If millions of auxotrophic cells containing a few prototrophs are placed on

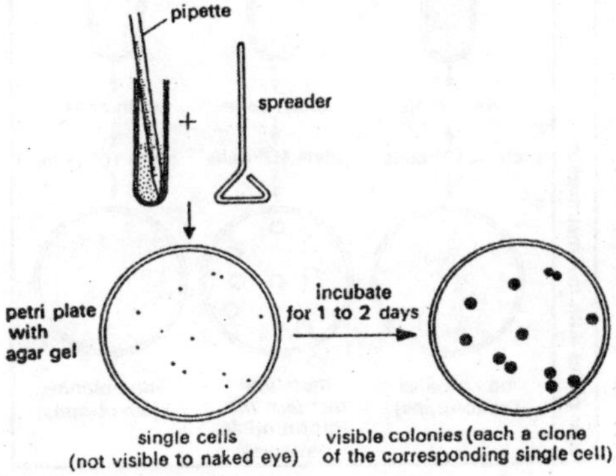

Technique of growing single cell bacterial colonies in the laboratory (spreader is used to spread a drop of suspension culture, on agar plate, giving single cells by repeated spreading).

an agar plate with minimal medium, only the prototrophs will grow, so that if the number of cells plated is known, the relative proportion of prototrophs can be easily worked out.

Discovery of Gene Transfer: Lederberg and Tatum, in their experiment on sexuality in bacteria, utilised two strains of *Escherichia coli* with different nutritional requirements: (i) strain A could grow on a minimal medium supplemented with methionine and biotin—designated as $met^-bio^-thr^+leu^+thi^+$ and (ii) strain B could grow on a minimal medium supplemented with threonine, leucine and thiamine—designated as $met^+bio^+thr^-leu^-thr^-$. Among petri-plates, all with unsupple-mented minimal medium, some plates were plated with strain A, others with strain B and still others with a mixture of strain A and strain B, which had already been grown in a liquid

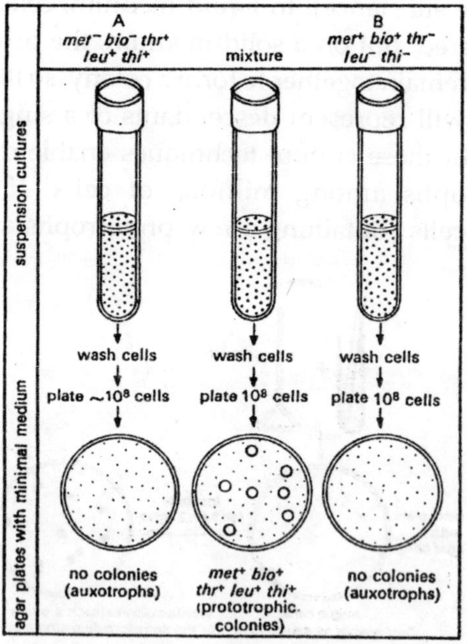

Demonstration of genetic recombination between bacterial cells as demonstrated by Lederberg and Tatum (note the presence of colonies only when the mixture of A and B is used for plating).

medium containing all the supplements (Fig.). The plates were incubated overnight and the following observation were made : (i) No colonies were formed on plates incubated either with strain A or with strain B. (ii) Few colonies (1 for every 10,000,000 cells plated, *i.e.*, with a frequency of 1×10^{-7}) were observed on plates incubated with a mixture of both the strains. This suggested that the prototrophs *($met^{+}bio^{+}thr^{+}leu^{+}thi^{+}$)* appeared due to recombination at a frequency of 1×10^{-7}.

Two questions on the above experiment could be raised : (i) Could the wild type colonies be produced due to mutations?, (ii) Could the growth of colonies be attributed to 'cross feeding' (leakage from one strain, of substances, which could be used by the other strain for growth) rather than genetic recombination.

The first question could be answered, because if wild type colonies were due to mutation, these should have appeared even on plates incubated with individual strains. Further, the strain being deficient for two or three genes, the possibility of simultaneous mutation in two or three genes would be very remote and therefore, could be ruled out. For the answer to the second question, another experiment was conducted, where a U tube was used, with such a filter that the pores were too small to allow the bacteria to pass, but will be large enough to allow the passage of fluid with the dissolved substances. Strain A was kept in one arm and strain B in the other arm (Fig.).

After they had been incubated for a few hours, the contents of each arm were separately tested on minimal medium. None of them was found to grew on a minimal medium, suggesting that physical contact between strain A and strain B was necessary for the generation of wild type strains or prototrophs. In other words, gene transfer or genetic recombination involving physical contact was responsible for the appearance of prototrophs.

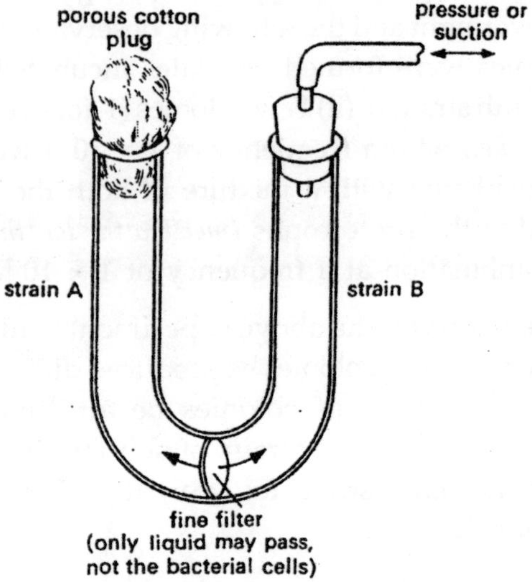

Experiment demonstrating the need of physical contact between bacteria, for genetic recombination to occur.

Discovery of Linkage in Bacteria: A simple two step experiment was performed by Lederberg and Tatum, using the above two strains (strain A = $met^{-}bio^{-}thr^{+}leu^{+}thi^{+}$ and strain B = $met^{+}bio^{+}thr^{-}leu^{-}thr^{-}$) to test whether or not the genes are organised into linkage group(s). In step one, a mixture of A and B was grown on a minimal medium supplemented with biotin so that both $met^{+}bio^{+}thr^{+}leu^{+}thi^{+}$ as well as $met^{+}bio^{-}thr^{+}leu^{+}thi^{+}$ could grow. They were designated as $met^{+}bio^{?}thr^{+}leu^{+}th^{+}$.

In step two, the colonies grown on biotin supplemented medium were tested on minimal medium (deficient for biotin) and were classified into two categories (*bio*+ and *bio*⁻). Similar tests were performed with other supplements (threonine, leucine and thiamine) also and the results are presented in Table, which suggests linkage, because in the absence linkage, due to independent assortment, 1 : 1 ratio between + and – strains for each supplement should be obtained.

Allele Frequencies in a Cross A x B as Observed by Lederberg and Tatum

A : $met^-bio^-thr^+leu^+tht^+$

B : $met^+bio^+thr^-liu^-thi^-$

Medium supplement	*Genotype of surviving colonies*	*Allelic frequencies at the unselected (?) locus*	
		+	–
1. Biotin	$met^+bio^?thr^+leu^+thi^+$	60	10
2. Threonine	$met^+bio^+thr^?leu^+thi^+$	37	9
3. Leucine	$met^+bio^+thr^+leu^?thi^+$	51	5
4. Thiamine	$met^+bio^+thr^+leu^+thi^?$	8	79

Donor (F^+ or Hfr) and Recipient (F^-) strains (Discovery of Fertility Factor or Sex Factor F): Among the above strain A *($met^-bio^-thr^+leu^+thi^+$)* and strain B *($met^+bio^+thr^-leu^-thr^-$)*, undergoing recombination, it was possible to designate them as donor and recipient strains on the basis of the following simple experiments involving treatment of either A or B with streptomycin (which does not kill immediately, but prevents cell division). When strain A was treated with streptomycin and mixed with strain B after washing out streptomycin, the frequency of colonies on minimal medium equalled those in control, where both strains were untreated.

On the other hand, when only strain B was similarly treated, no colonies were observed, suggesting that for recombination, cell division in strain B, but not in strain A, was essential. This suggested that gene transfer in *E. coli* is non-reciprocal and that one strain (A) is donor and the other (B) is recipient, which has to undergo cell division to form colonies after receiving genes from the donor strain (A). This differs from sexual reproduction where two parents contribute genetic material to an entirely new organism, the parents themselves remaining unaltered. Later on, through a series of experiments, it could be proved that the donor attribute of a strain is due to a transmissible fertility factor, F, which is absent in the recipient strain.

Therefore, the donor was designated as F^+ and recipient as F^-. It was also shown that although a F^+ strain can also act as a recipient, but F^- can not act as a donor unless it changes to F^+ through conjugation with a F^+ strain.

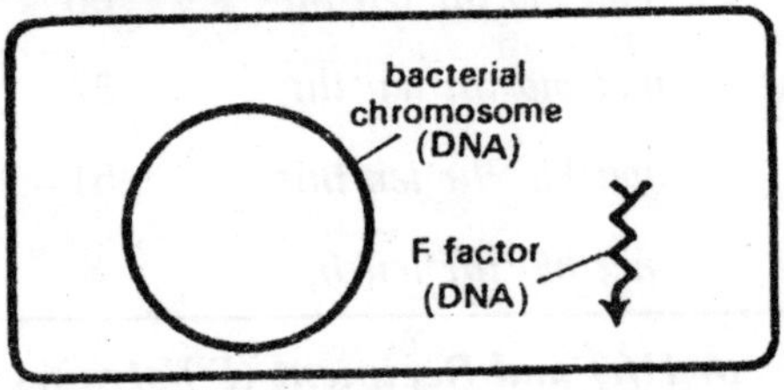

A bacterial cell showing circular DNA and F factor.

The F factor is composed of a circular DNA molecule of molecular weight 250,000 (about 1/40th of bacterial chromosome). Ordinarily only one F factor is found per cell (Fig.), which replicates with each cell division. A donor cell or F^+ can transmit F factor to recipient or F^- cells which in turn become donor or F^+ cells. This transmission of F factor is independent of transmission of chromosomal genes, so that in many cases F factor may be transmitted in high frequency while chromosomal genes are transmitted in a very low frequency (one per million cells).

However, rarely from F^+ populations, specific donor strains capable of transmitting chromosomal genes in high frequency (a thousand times that of F^+), could be isolated. These were called high frequency recombinants and designated as Hfr strains. Besides, higher frequency of recombination in Hfr, there is another important difference between F^+ and Hfr strains. The initial transfer of genes from a Hfr to a F^- strain was not

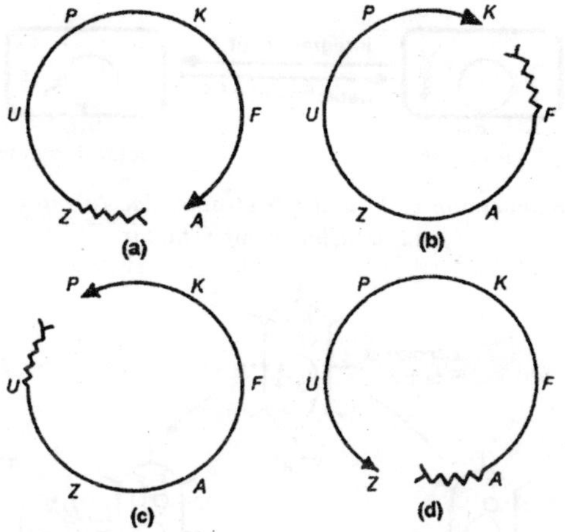

(A, B, C, D), Four hypothetical Hfr strains having different genes at their proximal ends.

strains of Hfr *E. coli*	order in which genes enter recipient cell
1	← A B C D E F G H I J K L M N O P
2	← D E F G H I J K L M N O P A B C
3	← F E D C B A P O N M L K J I H G
4	← I H G F E D C B A P O N M L K J
5	← M N O P A B C D E F G H I J K L

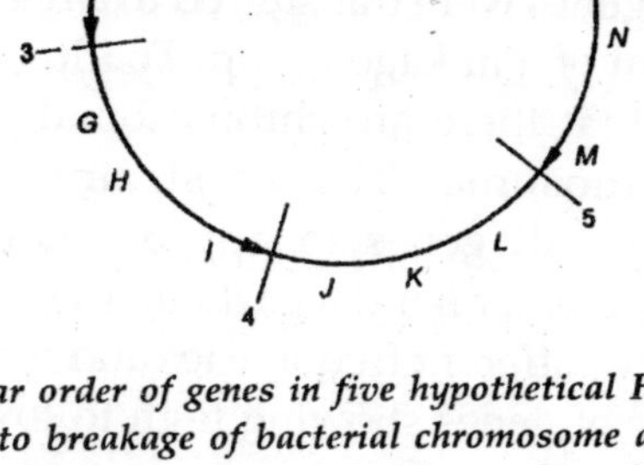

The linear order of genes in five hypothetical Hfr strains, resulting due to breakage of bacterial chromosome at different sites and subsequent orientation acquired by the resulting linear chromosome.

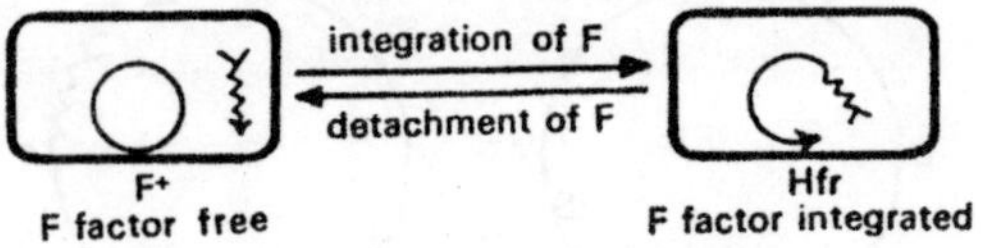

Interconversion of F+ and Hfr strains, due to integration and detachment of F factor.

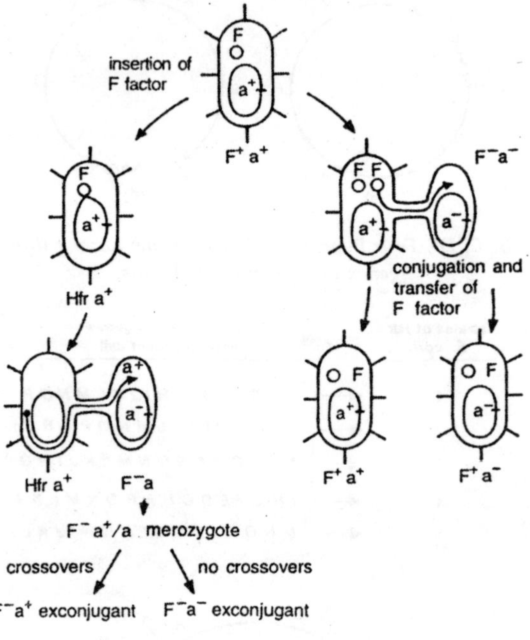

Sexual conjugation, showing two alternatives. In one case (right) the F factor remains free, while in the other case (left) the F factor gets attached to form Hfr.

random but the genes were transferred in a regular and defined order in the form of a linkage group. To illustrate this further, let us suppose that there are chromosomal genes *A* to *Z* on bacterial chromosome. The F^+ strains could produce recombinants for all genes in approximately equally low frequency. On the other hand a particular Hfr strain, transmits different genes in different frequencies and for a particular Hfr strain, the order of genes showing high to low recombination values is fixed.

However, the order of genes showing high to low recombination values differs in different Hfr strains so that while in one Hfr strain, *A* may show the highest recombination value, in other strains *K* or *P* or Z may show highest recombination (Fig.). But once the gene showing highest frequency is known, the order in which other genes will be transferred, can be easily predicted as shown in Figure. Moreover, while most of the F^- conjugating with F^+, become F^+, only very rarely F^- conjugating with Hfr would become F^+ or Hfr. It has also been shown that the F factor remains free in the cytoplasm in F^+ strains but remains integrated with the chromosome in Hfr strains. The position at which the F factor will be attached to chromosome differs in different Hfr strains. Also F^+ can become Hfr due to integration of F factor to the chromosome and *vice-versa* (Fig.).

When conjugation occurs between F^+ donor and F^- recipient, two possibilities exist (Fig.) (i) F factor may remain free in cytoplasm, so that only F factor will enter the recipient cell converting the recipient F^- into a donor F^+. (ii) F factor may get integrated and would thus make the distal part of bacterial chromosome. In this case the chromosome will become linear and would have a directional orientation, so that it would enter the recipient cell from the end away from attached F factor.

From the above discussion, it also emerges that the low recombination attribute of F^+ strain is due to presence of Hfr among F^+ cells in low frequency. When same Hfr is found in a relatively pure state, recombination frequency increases. In other words, for recombination to take place, F factor must be attached to bacterial chromosome and the circular chromosome should take up a linear orientation.

Conversion of F^+ into Hfr Strain: It has been shown that like the bacterial chromosome, fertility factor F is also circular, so that a crossover between the two rings would produce a larger ring with F inserted. The F is believed to consist of three regions: (i) origin, (ii) fertility genes and (iii) pairing region. The pairing region of F has homology with several region of bacterial chromosome, so that crossing over can take place at any one of these regions, producing different Hfr strains.

Fertility Factor F′ and Sexduction: During experiments with Hfr strains, initially (in 1959) an Hfr strain was found, which kept on producing F^+ cells at high frequencies. The fertility factor involved in this process was described as *F′* to distinguish it from normal F, due to following attributes: (i) F′-bearing F^+ strains often reverted back to an Hfr strain; (ii) *F′* always integrated at the same location to give the same original Hfr (not the different Hfr strains having different proximal and distal genes, as is usually observed). The origin of F′ was resolved through the following interesting observations. From a Hfr *lac*⁺ (with *lac*⁺ at distal end), an F^+ strain was derived, which transferred *lac*⁺ to *F⁻lac⁻* at a high frequency and *F⁻lac⁻* became F^+ *lac*⁺, which was shown to be

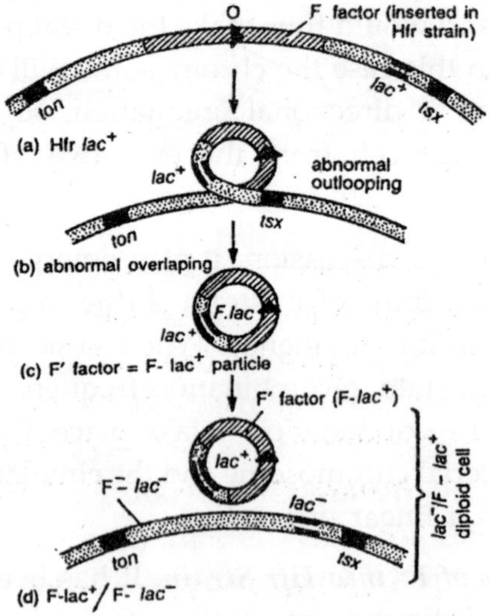

Origin of F′ factor (or F-lac) due to abnormal outlooping (a-c) and reintegration of F-lac⁺ into F⁻lac⁻ strain.

(*F-lac*$^+$/*lac*$^-$ (*lac*$^+$ carried F, so that in this case F′ = *F-lac*$^+$). Such F$^+$ strains with F′ are actually partial diploids or merozygotes. The use of F′ elements to create partial diploids is called sexduction or F-duction.

The origin of *F′* is shown in Figure, and may involve F′ carrying up to one quarter of the bacterial chromosome. These merozygotes carrying F′ have been used for recombination studies.

Mechanism of Chromosome Transfer: If the Hfr or F$^+$ donates its chromosome to F$^-$ during conjugation, the donor should actually die after conjugation. But this does not happen. There is evidence that Hfr chromosome replicates shortly before or during conjugation and only one of the two strands is transferred to F$^-$ cell and gets replicated there. This leaves a complete chromosome in Hfr or F$^+$ even after conjugation (Fig.).

Physical Structures Involved in Chromosome Transfer: The above transfer of chromosome is achieved through the conjugation tubes or F pili (singular pilus) protruding from cell walls of F$^+$ or Hfr cells. These pili are absent in F$^-$ cells, and come in contact with these *F*$^-$ cells to provide the passage for transfer. The pili have actually been observed under electron microscope.

Retrotransfer and Sexual Combination

Conjugation, as discussed above, assumed unidirectional transfer of genetic material from the donor to the recipient. In mid-1980's this unidirectional model was questioned when it was shown that genes can also be transferred in the opposite direction, *i.e.*, from recipient to the donor strain. This transfer of genes from recipient to the donor strain was described as retrotransfer, and was shown to be facilitated by the presence of plasmids like IncPl, IncM and IncN, which mediated 'back transfer' or 'back mobilisation'. There were other groups with plasmids like IncW, which could not mediate such a 'back transfer'. Subsequently, such a retrotransfer was shown to take place at a very high frequency, which was sometimes at least as frequent as the transfer of donor markers to recipients.

Transfer of genetic material in conjugation and retrotransfer can be one step (unidirectional) or two step (bidirectional) process. For instance, if Tra^+ Mob^- and Tra^-Mob^+. are the conjugating cells, the former being the donor and the latter recipient, then in theory, the transfer of Tra^- from recipient to doner and Tra^+ from donor the recipient can occur concurrently. This is a biderectional model or one step model of retrotransfer in contrast to the unidirectional or two step model in which the first step involves transfer of Tra^+ from donor to the recipient and the second step involves transfer of Tra^- from the recipient to the donor. There is strong support in favour of unidirectional model, thus vindicating the long-standing doctrine of unidirectional transfer in conjugation, although this transfer can take place in both the directions, one mediated by F factor and the other by certain plasmids.

Exeterial Mapping

Conjugation Mapping Through Interrupted Mating: In conjugation experiments, it was observed that the number of genes transmitted from donor to recipient was directly proportional to the time interval for which conjugation was allowed. Based on this feature, a technique called 'interrupted mating technique' was developed for mapping the bacterial chromosome. In this technique donor Hfr and recipient F^- strains are mixed and allowed to conjugate for a short period of time. Then samples are removed at periodic intervals and subjected to violent agitation to break the conjugation tube. The length of donor chromosome transmitted could then be determined and mapped in terms of time units required for transfer. It is known that 8 minutes are needed for conjugation to begin and then chromosome is transferred slowly in terms of time units (Fig.), one time unit being equal to one minute. The complete chromosome of *E. coli* is transferred in about 89 minutes (Fig.) and therefore the bacterial chromosome is 89 time units in length.

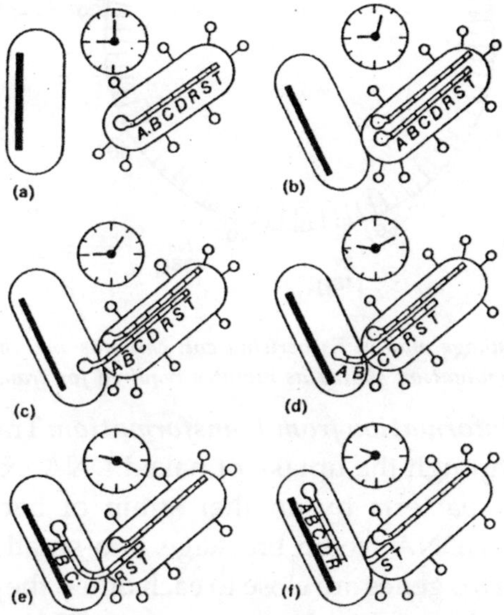

The transfer of genes in linear order from male bacterium (tagged with virus) to female; the length of transferred segment is dependent upon the time taken for transfer and the chromosome is, therefore, mapped in terms of time units.

When linkage maps in bacteria were prepared using several Hfr strains, these maps differed with respect to the first and the last genes of the map. However, once we know the first gene transferred and the direction of transfer of subsequent genes, the order is predetermined as shown in hypothetical cases used in Figure. The only way these results could be explained, was through the assumption of a circular map, which cleaves at any point due to attachment of F factor to form a linear chromosome that enters the recipient cell. Circular nature of linkage group was later confirmed by evidence for physical circular nature of bacterial chromosome.

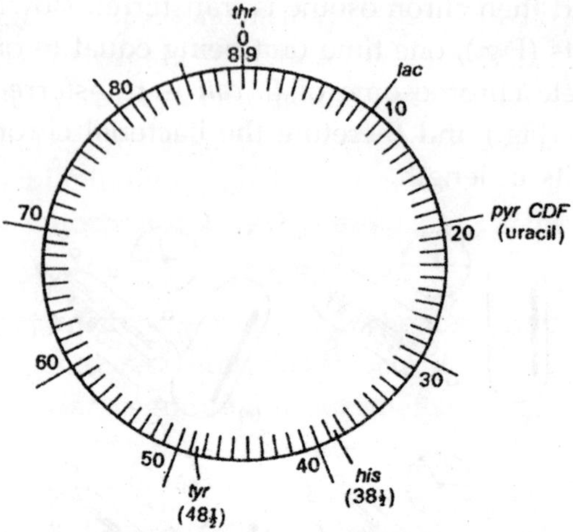

Circular linkage map of Escherichia coli chromosome, the units of recombination shown as minutes required for transfer.

Linkage Information from Transformation: Transformation is achieved through the uptake of naked DNA extracted from one strain of bacteria by another strain of bacteria. While extracting this DNA, some breakage into small pieces does take place. If two genes are close to each other, they have better chance of being carried on the same piece of DNA, thus causing double transformation.

Similarly, genes widely separated, will have a better chance of being carried on separate DNA segments and the frequency of double transformation will be the product of single transformation frequencies. A departure from product rule of probability for the observed frequency of double recombinants will prove close linkage.

Recombination After Gene Transfer: When a chromosome segment is transferred from a donor to a recipient strain (or through transduction or transformation), this transferred segment must be integrated into host genome by an exchange mechanism to produce a stable recombinant. The recipient cell at this stage is called a merozygote (partial diploid) which has the complete genome of F^-, called endogenote and an incomplete genome called exogenote derived from F^+ or Hfr. An even number of crossovers, rather than a single or odd number of crossovers, allows incorporation of a part of the genome from exogenote into the endogenote; one of the two products of exchange (*i.e.*, a linear fragment) is usually lost (Fig.).

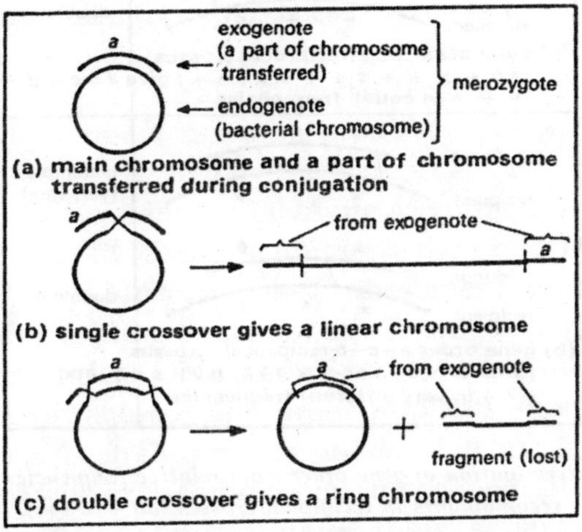

Recombination in bacteria after gene transfer (single and double crossovers give linear and ring chromosomes respectively).

High Resolution Mapping: Interrupted mating technique described earlier allows only low resolution mapping. For high resolution mapping within a distance of 2 minutes, the interrupted mating is not useful, and we need to study the stable recombinants, rather than the genes transferred. For example if ade^+ and *leu+ arc* the two genes transferred, we can work out frequencies of colonies with leu^+ and leu^- among those with ade^+ (if ade^+ is more frequent than leu^+). The proportion of leu^- (ade^+ leu^-) among total ade^+, *i.e.*, $\{(ade^+\ leu^+)+(ade^+\ leu^-)\}$, will give the recombination distance between ade^+ and leu^+.

$$\text{Recomb. } (ade\text{–}leu) = \frac{(ade^+ leu^-)}{(ade^+ leu^+) + (ade^+ leu^-)}$$

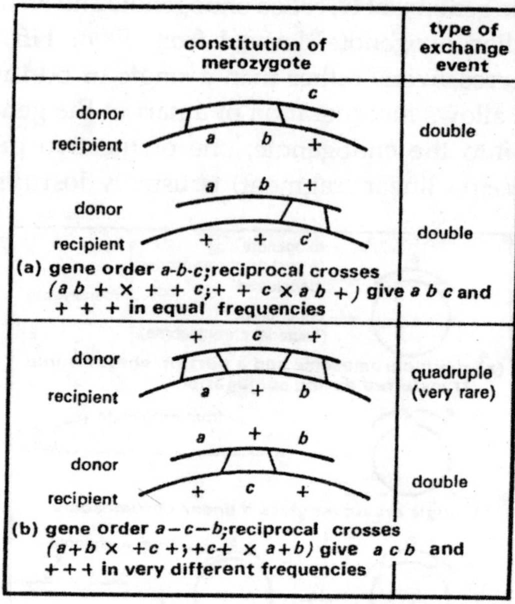

Determination of gene order from relative frequencies of recombinants in reciprocal crosses (ab + × ++c).

It has been shown that 1 minute on the map is equal to 20 per cent recombination, calculated as above.

Linear Order of Genes: If two genes are very close *(b* and *c)* with respect to a third gene *(a),* then it becomes difficult to determine the gene order *(a–b–c* or *a–c–b),* because the recombination frequencies between *a* and *b* and between *a* and *c* will be similar. This can be resolved by using reciprocal crosses: abc^+ (Hfr) x a^+b^+c (F^-) and a^+b^+c (Hfr) × abc^+ (F^-). In this case prototrophs *(*a^+ b^+ c^+*)* and the mutants *(abc)* will result in equal frequencies from two reciprocal crosses if the gene order is *a–b–c* and they will be produced in dramatically different frequencies, if the gene order is *a–c–b* (Fig.).

Sporulation and Cell Division in Bacteria: Bacterial cell division and associated chromosome segregation were earlier considered to be passive processes. The chromosome separation was believed to be followed by a mere constriction in the elongated cell, resulting into two daughter cells. This picture has been completely overturned, in view of recent advances, which demonstrated the presence of centromere like structures and mitosis like machinery for cell division in bacteria. Several genes involved in chromosome segregation in bacteria have now been identified and their functions elucidated.

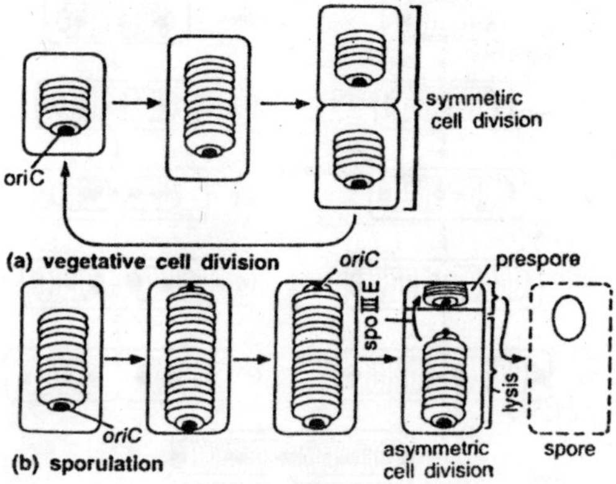

Asymmetric cell division during sporulation of Bacillus subtilis.

Asymmetric Cell Division during Sporulation in Bacillus Subtilis: In *B. subtilis,* sporulation occurs at the time of starvation (no sporulation occurs in *E. coli),* and involves an asymmetric division of the cell. It involves transfer of one third of a chromosome into the smaller cell, leaving about two-third of the chromosome in the mother cell.

The DNA transferred to the smaller cell or prespore consists of 500 kb of the origin of DNA replication *(oriC). A* protein SpoIIIE then helps in the transfer of the remaining DNA from the mother cell into the prespore, possibly through a pore in the septum, and the mother cell lyses, releasing the mature dormant spore (Fig.). This observation, along with the other experimental results obtained from the division of vegetative cells of *B. subtilis* and *E. coli* suggested that *oriC* regions of the two chromosomes in the dividing cell of *B. subtilis* are located close to two poles and the *ter*C region is near the midpoint of the cell. A protein SpoJ/ParB binds at or near the *ori*C region, and helps in cell division.

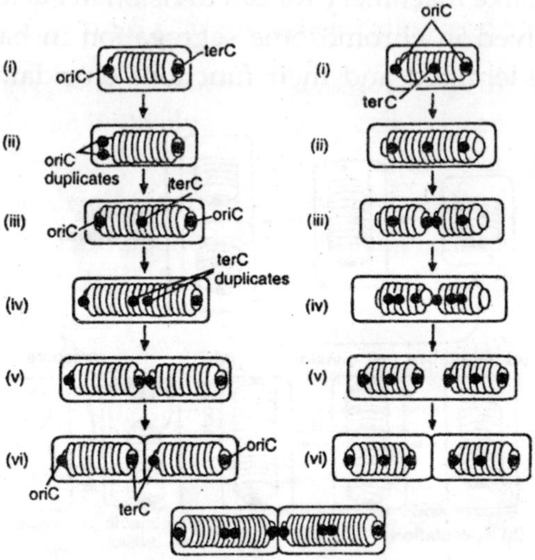

Segregation of chromosomes during vegetative cell division in (a) E. coli and (b) B. subtilis.

Vegetative Cell Division in E. Coli and B. Subtilis

Chromosome Segregation: Chromosome segregation during bacterial cell division is an active process and involves two different patterns of movements, (i) In *E. coli,* there is a single *ori*C, near one pole of the cell, and a *ter*C near the other pole. After duplication, one of the two daughter *ori*C moves from one pole to the other, and *ter*C moves towards the mid-cell and gets duplicated there, (ii) In *B. subtilis* cells, there are two *ori*C at the two poles and one *ter*C near the middle of the cell. Each *ori*C after moving to a position between the pole and *ter*C divides and the sister foci move away from each other to occupy two poles of a daughter cell; *ter*C also duplicates and occupies mid-cell positions in each of the two daughter nucleoids (Fig.).

The movement of *oriC*, after duplication may also involve action of some kind of spindle apparatus and 'motor proteins'. The genes spoJ and smc in *B. subtilis* and mukB in *E. coli* may encode proteins, that might play a role comparable to that of spindle and motor proteins.

Septum Formation: At the time of *E. coli* cell division, several proteins, including FtsZ, assemble in the middle of the cell. FtsZ was shown to form a ring like structure, much before the constriction is initiated. Other cell division proteins that are recruited later, include products of three genes: *minC*, *minD* and *minE*.

The mutations in these genes give 'minicell-producing (min) mutants', which divide not at the middle, but at the pole giving daughter cells, which are 1/4th (mini cells) and 3/4th (bigger) of the parent cell. Protein MinC is a division inhibitor, MinD (having ATPase activity) stimulates MinC activity and MinE ensures medial cell division, by inhibiting MinC-MinD interaction. Consequently, in the absence of MinE, MinCD prevents formation of the FtsZ ring in the middle of the cell. Following steps are involved in the septum formation in *E. coli* (Fig.). (i) MinE-GFP (GFP=green fluorescent protein) forms a ring like structure at the middle of the cell, preventing MinCD inhibitory activity at the site and allows later the assembly of FtsZ ring in the middle. (ii) MinCD (a division inhibitor) accumulates alternately (every 10-30 seconds) at the membrane periphery on either side of MinE ring; in between polar shifts, the protein appears to desiccate from the membrane periphery to accumulate in the cytoplasm; this disallows formation of FtsZ ring at 1/4 or 3/4 sites in the two cell halves. (iii) Additional cell division proteins are recruited to the FtsZ ring, resulting in septum formation. (iv) MinE ring disassembles before completion of constriction and septum formation.

In *B. subtilis*, homologues of MinC and MinD are available, but MinE is absent and replaced by DivIVA, so that MinCD-

DivIVA in *B subtilis,* like Min CDE system of *E. coli,* acts at the level of FtsZ. However, the mechanism of action of DivIVA protein in *B. subtilis* differs from that of MinE protein in *E. coli.* DivIVA-GFP localises to both cell poles, and later also appears in the middle of the cell.

Sequestration of MinCD inhibitor to the poles, allows assembly of FtsZ ring in the middle. DivIVA and MinCD are now recruited to the middle and constriction is initiated. FtsZ is disassembled as soon as the constriction is complete, but DivIVA and MinCD remain at the newly formed poles, preventing further division at these polar sites (Fig.).

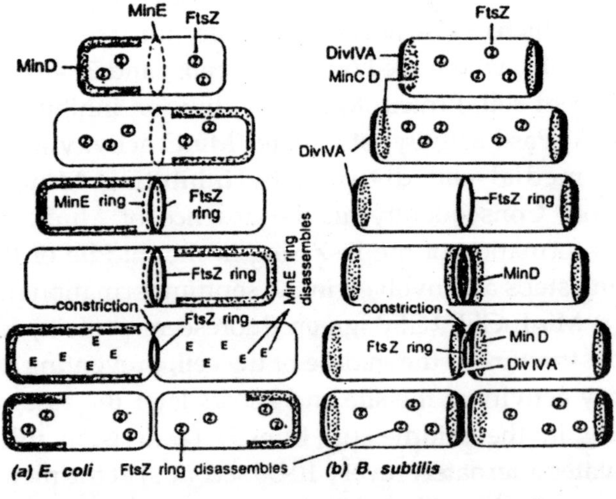

Septum formation during vegetative cell division in (a) E. coli and (b) B. subtilis.

Replication and Recombination in Viruses: Viruses can produce copies of themselves within the host cells, and can change through mutations. Depending upon the host which a virus infects, these can be broadly placed in three categories : (i) animal viruses, (ii) plant viruses and (iii) bacterial viruses or bacteriophages. Simplest of these three classes are bacteriophages, which have been most extensively utilised for study of genetics of viruses. Genetic recombination was also demonstrated between different strains of bacteriophages by M. Delbruck, W.T. Bailey and A.D. Hershey. These workers were also able to detect and artificially induce mutations in these organisms. Drs. A.D. Hershey, M. Delbruck and S.E. Luria shared Nobel Prize in medicine for the year 1969, for their contribution to replication and recombination in viruses.

Replication of Bacteriophages: A typical bacteriophage (abbreviated as 'phage' meaning 'eaters of bacteria') consists of a head with protein sheath containing DNA and a tail with tail fibres (Fig.). After infection, phage DNA forces the host to work for the parasite, so that complete host machinery is utilised for replication of phage particle.

The infected cell thus produces new protein subunits for the phage head and tail and also makes additional DNA segments identical to DNA of the invading phage particle. In this manner, a bacterial cell that has been infected by phage will undergo lysis (breaks open) within about 30 minutes and will release about 100 phage particles complete in all respects (Fig.).

Lysogenic Bacteria: The bacteriophages which cause lysis of bacterial cells (as described above) are called 'virulent' phages. There are other phages called 'temperate' phages, which may either cause lysis like virulent phages do, or may attach to bacterial chromosome thus forming its integral part (Fig.).

In the latter case, phage DNA would replicate only when bacterial chromosome replicates and will stay there as a symbiont rather than as a parasite. In this state virus is called 'provirus', and infected bacteria are called lysogenic, which means that the bacterial cell contains a property which can cause lysis. When lysogenic bacteria are exposed to ultraviolet light or X-rays or active chemicals like nitrogen mustard or organic peroxide, the temperate virus assumes a virulent state (Fig.).

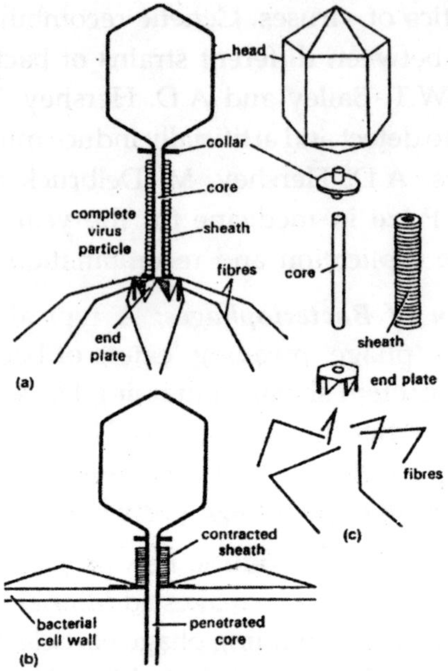

T4 bacteriophage and its components: (a) on top left-a complex phage particle is shown; (b) on bottom left-a phage particle attached to bacterial cell wall is shown; (c) on the right-various components, are shown.

Particles like temperate phages, which can remain in integrated as well as in free state within a cell are dispensable elements and are called 'episomes'. The sex factor or F factor earlier described in this chapter.

Transduction: When certain proviruses turn into virulent viruses thereby causing lysis of host cell, they may carry with them segments of host's DNA. If such virus particles carrying a segment of DNA from one host infects another host which is different than the first one, the latter may inherit some of the properties of the former host due to transfer of DNA segment through infecting phage (Fig.). This phenomenon of transfer of genetic material from one bacterial strain to another through the agency of virus is called transduction and was discovered in 1952 by N.D. Zinder and J. Lederberg at the University of Wisconsin, U.S.A.

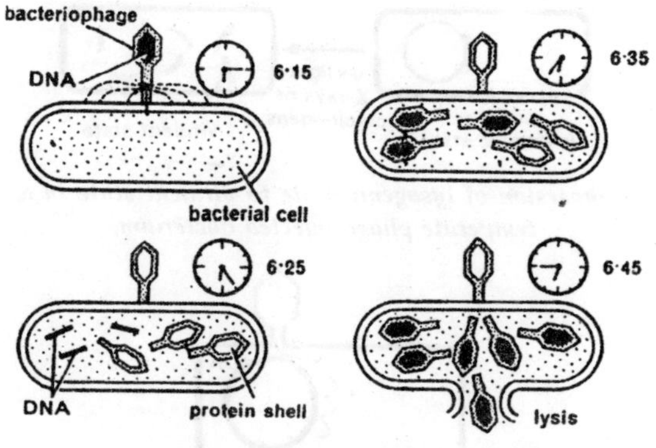

Different stages of infection, multiplication and lysis of virus particles in a bacterial cell; the clock shows the time taken for different steps of reproduction of virus.

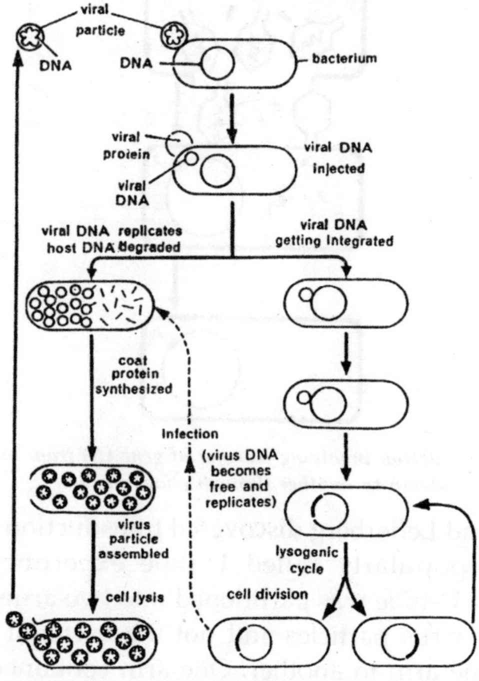

The life cycle of temperate phages, showing two patterns: (a) on the left is shown the virulent state and, (b) on the right is shown the lysogenic state, where the virus particle attaches to bacterial chromosome, but may become free and virulent at a later stage.

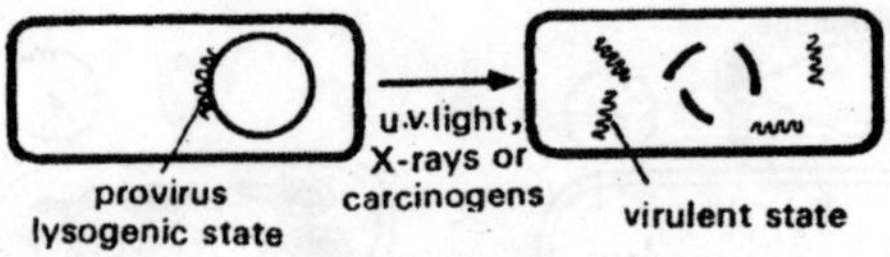

Conversion of lysogenic state to virulent state in a temperate phage infected bacterium.

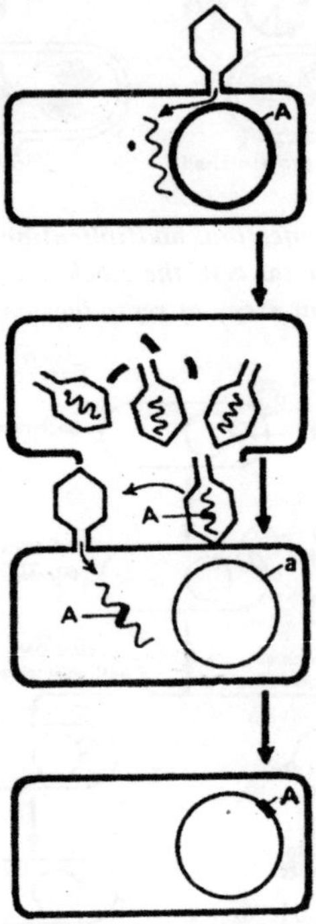

Transduction involving transfer of gene* (A) *from one strain to another through phage particle.

Zinder and Lederberg discovered transduction through an experiment popularly called U-tube experiment. In this experiment a U-tube was partitioned into two arms by a filter, so that only virus particles and not the bacterial cells could pass from one arm to another. One arm contained lysogenic bacteria carrying latent virus and the other arm contained bacteria susceptible to this virus. Rarely lysogenic bacteria could undergo lysis and release virus particles which crossed the filter and infected the other susceptible strain, which got destroyed releasing virus particles. These released particles carried genetic material from susceptible strain and through the filter again reached the lysogenic strain and transferred the genetic material to this lysogenic strain. Since two bacterial strains could not come in contact, no conjugation was possible. An enzyme was also used which destroyed free DNA, so that the possibility of transformation was also eliminated (Fig.).

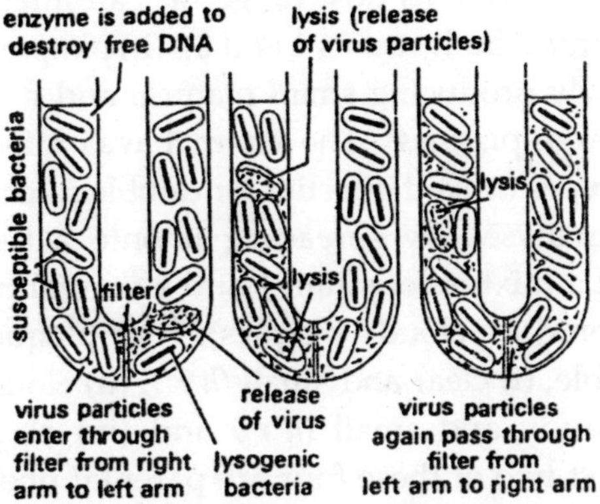

The U-tube experiment of Zinder and Lederberg showing the transfer of genetic material from one strain of bacterium to another through the agency of a bacteriophage (transduction).

Recombination in Viruses: Viruses can undergo recombination in host cells. For instance if two strains of a virus having genotypes a^+b^- and a^-b^+ are allowed to infect the same host cell, the resulting progeny of virus will also have recombinants a^+b^+ and a^-b^-, in addition to parental combinations a^+b^- and a^-b^+. The phenomenon of recombination in viruses was described for the first time by A.D. Hershey and R. Rotman in 1949 and has been utilised for preparing linkage maps of viruses. Linkage maps in T_2 and T_4 phages have been found to be circular, as is the case in *Escherichia coli* chromosome.

Circular Genetic Maps in Viruses: The viruses, being very small particles, are often considered not suitable for inheritance studies due to non-availability of scorable traits. However, plaque morphology (large vs. small, fuzzy vs. sharp), host range and virulence are characteristic features of bacteriophages (plaque = clear area produced on opaque lawn of bacteria on the surface of a dish of solid medium), which have been used for inheritance and recombination studies.

Inheritance and recombination in viruses can be illustrated by a cross in T_2 phage, attempted by Alfred Hershey. This cross ($h^-r^+ \times h^+r^-$) involved: (i) host range (h^+ can infect only strain 1 and h^- can infect both strains 1 and 2); (ii) plaque morphology (r^+ lyses slowly producing small plaques and r^- lyses rapidly producing large plaques). The strain 1 was infected by both phage genotypes (mixed infection or double infection) and the lysate was analysed by spreading it onto a bacterial lawn composed of a mixture of strain 1 and 2 (h^- will produce clear and h^+ will produce cloudy plaques). Four plaque types were distinguishable: (i) clear and small (h^-r^+), (ii) cloudy and large (h^+r), (iii) cloudy and small (h^+r^+) and (iv) clear and large (h^-r^-). The first two of these four are parental phenotypes and the last two are recombinants, so that the recombination frequency (RF) can be calculated as follows:

$$RF = \frac{(h^+r^-) + (h^-r^-)}{\text{total plaques}}$$

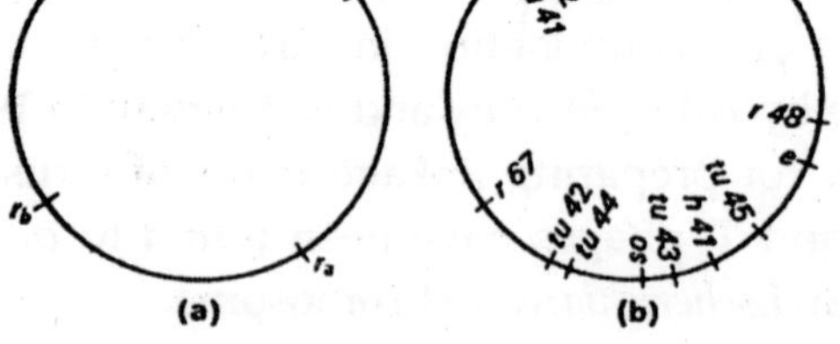

(a) Circular genetic map of T2 phage, showing only four genes, (b) Circular genetic map of T4 phage; h = host range; ac = acridine resistance; tu = turbid plaques; os = resistance to osmotic shock; e = lysis defective; r = rough plaques.

In order to prepare the linkage map, several rapid-lysis genotypes (*r1, r2, r3,* in order of discovery) were available and the corresponding strains were called r_a, r_b and r_c. Utilizing these three strains with h^+ and h^- genotypes, following crosses were made: (i) $r_a^- h^+ \times r_a^+ h^-$; (ii) $r_b^- h^+ \times r_b^+ h^-$; (iii) $r_c^- h^+ \times r_c^+ h^-$; (iv) $r_c^- r_b^+ \times r_c^+ r_b^-$. The recombination frequencies were calculated and following two equally probable linear orders were available: $r_a – r_c – h – r_b$ and $r_c – h – r_b – r_a$. This can be explained only if the circular map shown in Figure is accepted. This gives evidence for a circular genetic map for a T-even (T_2 or T_4) phage.

Recombination in T_4 phage has also been studied by S. Benzer resolving the fine structure of *rII* locus.

11

Product of Genes

Some proteins in the cell are required in small quantities, but others may be required in large quantities, so that the demands can not be easily met. These demands can be met in either of the following two ways:

(i) In some cases, a solitary gene is present in the cell but is transcribed repeatedly to produce large number of messenger RNA molecules and these mRNA molecules act as templates for many rounds of protein synthesis. For instance, although the gene coding for silkworm protein fibroin is present in only one copy per haploid complement, but it keeps on making silk actively. Similarly in a cell engaged in exclusive synthesis of haemoglobin, a solitary copy of the gene produces large quantities of (α or β polypeptide chains of haemoglobin. However, although a whole family of related a globin genes are found in each cell, different but solitary *a* globin genes function at different stages of development (see later).

(ii) In other cases, multiple copies of a gene are found in the same cell, all taking part in transcription within a cell, giving rise to large quantities of the gene product as in case of ribosomal RNA (rRNA) genes, histone genes, tRNA genes, heat shock protein genes, SnRNA (small nuclear RNA) genes, actin genes, etc. It is these multi-gene families, which will make the subject of discussion in this chapter.

Family of Group-gene

A multi-gene family is a group of similar, but not necessarily identical sequences, each sequence representing a gene, so that the gene is present in multiple copies. These multi-gene families can be broadly classified in at least three groups:

(i) The different members of a multi-gene family, if not identical, may function in different tissues of the organism at a particular time, or in the same tissue at different times. A mechanism will be available for tissue specific or temporal (time specific) regulation of activity of different members of such a multi-gene family (*e.g.* globin genes).

(ii) In other cases all members of a multi-gene family may function in a specific tissue or at a specific time, but all members will function in the same cell due to heavy demand for the gene product, as in case of heat shock genes expressed on heat shock, or storage protein genes expressed during seed formation.

(iii) In still other cases, there may be multi-gene families, members of which will ordinarily function in all living cells at all times as in case of rRNA genes or SnRNA genes.

How to Locate Multi-gene Families?: If cellular DNA, after digestion, is electrophoresed and hybridised with radioactively labelled rRNA or mRNA product of the gene sequence being analysed or even with a genomic or cDNA probe, the number of DNA-RNA or DNA-DNA hybrid molecules formed can be estimated by comparing them with those formed in case of single copy genes. This can be done by measurements of radioactivity in the hybrid molecules by any one of the different methods available.

The presence of multiple copies will suggest the presence of a multi-gene family. Some details of individual multi-gene families illustrating the above situations will be discussed in the following text.

Genes Function

Multi-gene Families with Divergent Members Globin Gene Family in Human Genome: Although in adult humans only single genes, each specifying a and b polypeptide chains of haemoglobin are expressed, this is not enough during development, such that a whole family of related a globin genes and another family of b globin genes function.

These genes are turned off and on in a coordinated and sequential manner during embryo development till the fetus is born, depending upon the intracellular milieu. The constitution of haemoglobins found at different stages of development are shown in Table and Figure.

The Constitution of Haemoglobins in Humans at different Stages of Development

Development stage	*Constitution of haemoglobin*
1. Embryonic (up to 8 weeks)	$\zeta_2\varepsilon_2, \zeta_2\gamma_2$ and $\alpha_2\varepsilon_2$
2. Fetal	$\alpha_2\gamma_2$
3. Adult	$\alpha_2\delta_2, \alpha_2\beta_2$

ζ, - zeta; α = alpha like chains; ε = epsilon;

β = beta like chains

During development, zeta (ζ is expressed first and is replaced later by α. In beta (β) pathway similarly epsilon (ε) and gamma (γ) are expressed first, which are later replaced by delta (δ) and beta (β). In the adult, $\alpha_2\beta_2$ forms 97% of the haemoglobin, $\alpha_2\delta_2$ forms 2% and $\alpha_2\gamma_2$ (fetal form) forms the remaining 1% due to persistence of the fetal form (Fig.).

In humans, α-like globin genes are located on chromosome 16 and β-like globin genes are located on chromosome 11

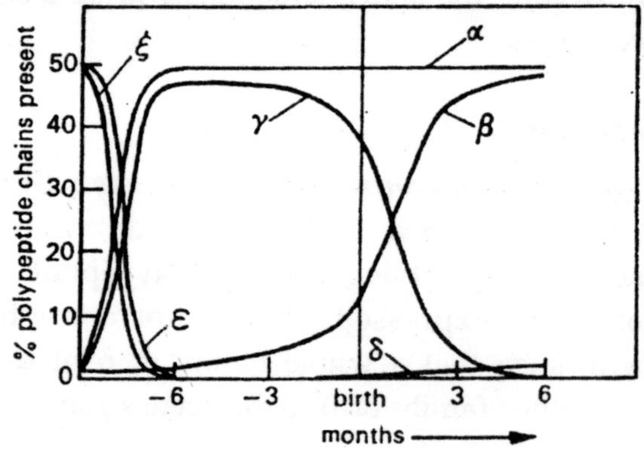

Temporal regulation of the synthesis of different polypeptides representing a and b" polypeptide chains of haemoglobin molecules during pregnancy and after birth in human beings.

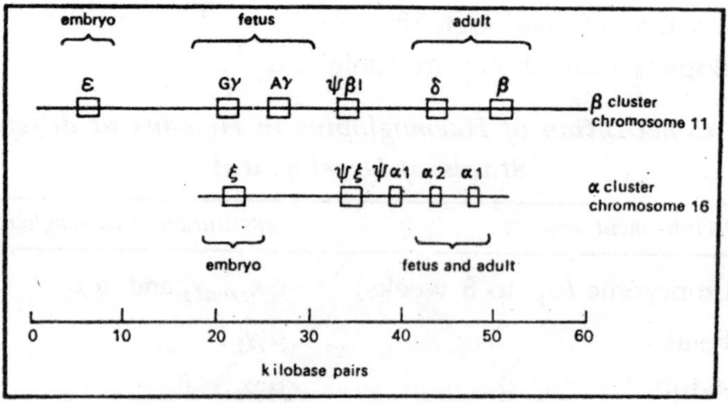

Arrangement of human β and α globin gene clusters on chromosomes 11 and 16.

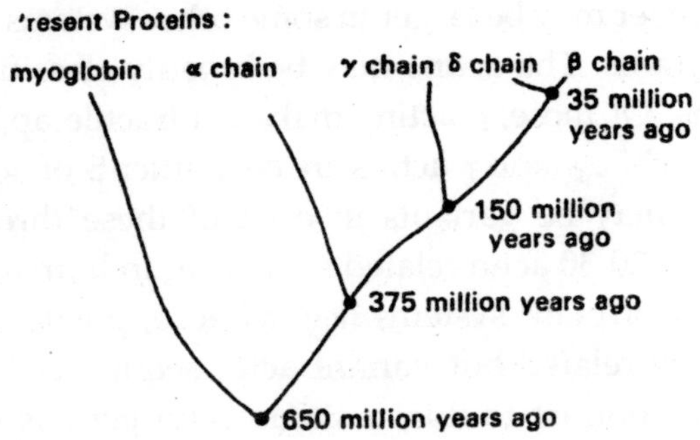

Phylogenetic relationships among myoglobin and four haemoglobin chains deduced from amino acid substitutions (redrawn from Zuckerkandl, Nature 192, 1961).

(Fig.). Between the genes are spacer regions (that are not transcribed) and are also present pseudogenes that are related to globin genes, but are never transcribed. The individual genes of globin gene family are arranged in the order in which they function during the development of fetus (Fig.), although in other families such an arrangement is not always necessary. It has been shown that in these sequences, the coding regions show little divergence, but spacers in between the genes show considerable diversity as is the case in many other families.

The only explanation for this is that the protein function puts a constraint on the evolution of coding sequence, while no such constraint is exercised in spacer region which is fast evolving. Based on the degree of similarity in the amino acid sequences of globin of different mammals, evolutionary trees have also been prepared in the past (Figs.).

Actin Gene Family in Eukaryotes: Actin genes represent a multi-gene family, where the members are homologous, but non-identical, giving rise to slightly different variants so that different members function either at different times in the same tissue or in different tissues at the same time.

For instance, a minimum of six closely related polypeptides are synthesised in different cells at different times in mammals and the number may be larger in some other systems including flowering plants. The actins may be broadly classified as α, β and γ actins. Of these, γ actins make contractile apparatus of the muscle, while β and γ actins are constituents of non-muscle cells. There may be variants in each of these three classes, making up to 20-30 actin related sequences in human genome. In a number of plant systems (*e.g.* tobacco, potato, etc.) also, more than 20 related but variant actin sequences have been reported. In contrast to this, a single actin gene is known in yeast.

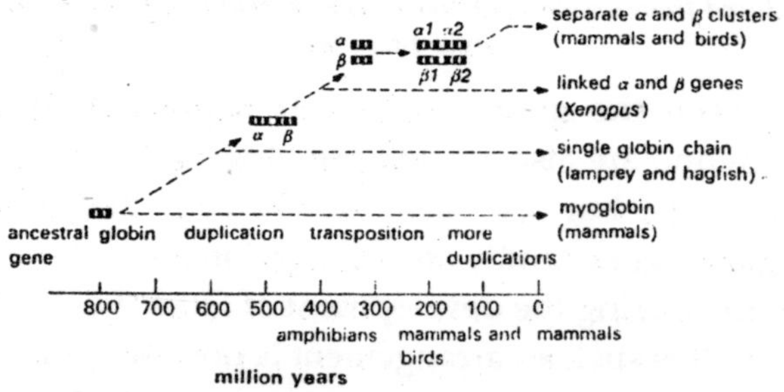

Myoglobin differentiation into a and p chains from earliest period in the history.

Other Multi-gene Families with Divergent Members: Other multi-gene families having divergent members, that have been studied include genes for the following:

(i) albumin and a fetoprotein (major components of blood plasma), serine proteases, the interferons (for defense against viral infection) and the immunoglobulins;

(ii) *chorion* proteins making the major component of egg shell in insects.

Multi-gene Families with Identical Genes

In some cases, in order to produce large quantities of a gene product, many copies of identical genes are required. These, genes may occur in the form of repeat units, each comprising of (i) a coding region, which is highly conserved to produce exactly the same gene product, and (ii) a spacer region, which may show divergence. Some examples of these multi-gene families will be described in this section.

Multiple Copies of Histone Genes: The five major histone proteins, namely H_1, H_2A, H_2B, H_3, H_4 are involved in the packing of DNA into nucleosome, the chromatin subunit. When DNA is duplicated during S phase of the cell cycle, large quantities of these histone proteins are needed. To meet this demand, for each of the histone genes, there are present (i) 10-20 copies in birds and mammals and (ii) 600-800 copies in sea urchin and newt (amphibians). A higher number in amphibians suggests a response to their need for rapid cell division. The five genes for five histones form a basic unit that is repeated, although different genes within a repeat unit may differ in orientation (Fig.). These genes (coding sequences) in a repeat unit are highly conserved, but the spacer region differs in different organisms. The histone genes differ from most other eukaryotic genes in having their transcripts devoid of introns and poly A tails.

Another interesting feature of the multi-gene family of histone genes observed in *Drosophila* is the presence of an 'attachment site' per repeat unit (Fig.), 100 such repeat units being present in each haploid genome. With the help of

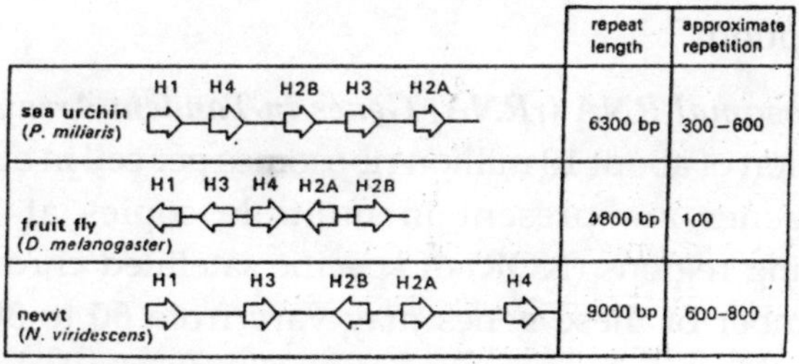

Organisation of highly repeated histone gene clusters in several organisms; genes are separated by non-transcribed spacer (NTS) regions; the direction of transcription is shown by arrows; the clusters are tandemly repeated in sea urchin and fruit fly, but not in the newt.

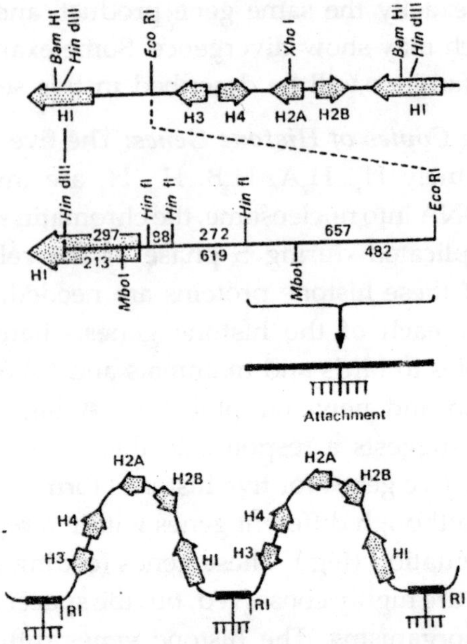

(a) A restriction map of major histone gene cluster in Drosophila; each repeat unit has one specific attachment site to the nuclear scaffold, this attachment site is HinI/Eco R I DNA segment, 657 bp long; (b) schematic representation showing how Drosophila histone repeats might be attached to the nuclear scaffold.

attachment site, the genes remain attached to nuclear scaffold (scaffold is the protein backbone of chromosomes, to which DNA remains attached). These attachment sites help in transcription.

Ribosomal RNA (rRNA) Genes in Tandem Arrays: For the production of about 10 million ribosomes per cell in eukaryotes, rRNA genes are present in multiple copies at nucleolar organizing regions (NOR) of specific satellited chromosomes. The number of these genes may vary from 50 to 30,000 in a cell and this number may be unequally distributed on NORs, if more than one such loci are present. The DNA comprising these genes is called rDNA (ribosomal DNA), which is repetitive in nature. Each repeat unit has:

(i) a coding region with genes that specify 18S, 5.8S and 28S rRNA molecules,

(ii) a spacer region called intergenic spacer (IGS) and

(iii) internal transcribed spacers (ITS) one each between 18S and 5.8S genes and between 5.8S and 28S genes.

Since parts of IGS region adjoining the coding region, known as external transcribed spacers (ETS), is also transcribed, the use of the term non-transcribed spacer (NTS) for the whole spacer region has been considered to be inappropriate. Actually, the NTS makes only a part of the IGS (Fig.), the remaining part of IGS being ETS. The IGS in its turn has a region consisting of a tandem array of variable number of subrepeats ranging from 100-300 bp (bp = base pairs) in length.

The variation in number and size of the subrepeats in IGS is responsible for variation in length of the repeat unit (IGS + coding region). The rDNA repeat units are usually looped off from the main chromosome fibre, in the form of extended threads at nucleolar organizing region. These loops, in association with specific proteins form the nucleoli, where rRNA synthesis and processing really takes place.

The number of nucleoli and, the corresponding number of nucleolar organizing (satellited) chromosomes in an organism may vary from one to several. At each locus (NOR), rDNA repeat units may evolve independently both in length and also in the nucleotide sequence of the spacer region, so that the length of the repeat unit 'including coding and spacer regions (non-transcribed spacer or NTS; external transcribed spacer or ETS and internal transcribed spacers or ITS) varies from about 7 kb (kilobase pairs) to 14 kb. In wheat and barley, it is usually 9 kb-10 kb (Fig.).

5S RNA Genes: 5S RNA genes are present independently of the rDNA which is localised at the NOR in eukaryotes (5S RNA is also found in ribosomes). However, in prokaryotes and yeast, 5S RNA genes are present in close vicinity of rDNA (Fig.). The 5S RNA genes are also organised in tandem repeats, each repeat consisting of a gene 120 bp long and a spacer region. The length of the complete repeat is 375 bp in *Drosophila*. In wheat, there are two loci for 5S RNA having repeats of different lengths, 480 bp and 500 bp. These repeat units may sometimes carry pseudogenes (instead of functional genes), which are not used for synthesis of any RNA.

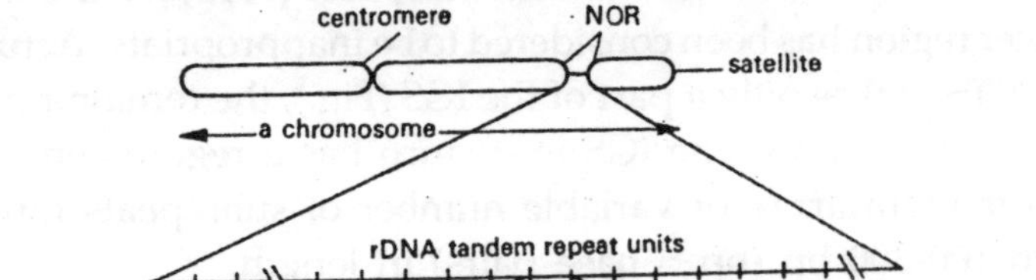

Organisation of ribosomal DNA (rDNA) in nucleolar organizing region (NOR) of a eukaryotic chromosome (IGS = intergenic spacer; NTS = non-transcribed spacer; ETS = external transcribed spacer; ITS = internal transcribed spacer; 18S, 5.8S, 26S = different genes responsible for I8S rRNA, 5.8S rRNA and 26S rRNA).

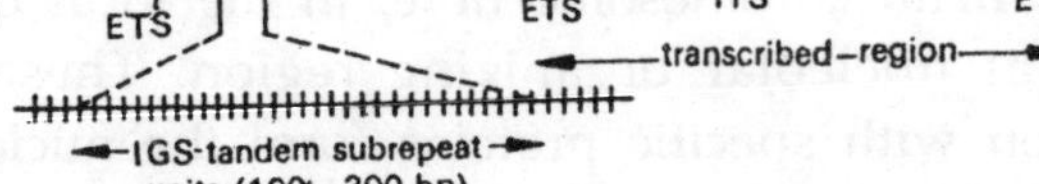

An outline of the structure of rDNA in wheat and barley.

tRNA Multi-gene Families: The genes for each of the different tRNAs are also found in multiple copies to meet the heavy demands of the cell for the production of tRNA molecules. Ten to several hundred genes for each tRNA are present in each haploid genome. While in some cases with fewer copies of a gene, these copies are dispersed, in other cases like *Xenopus* (a toad), tandem repeats of long sequences (each repeat having genes for several different tRNAs) are found. For instance, in *Xenopus,* a 3.2 kb repeat length has 8 genes, 2 for $tRNA_f^{met}$ and six others for six different tRNA molecules (Fig.). In still other cases (*e.g. Drosophila),* genes for completely different tRNA species are clustered over a length of several thousand base pairs. Sometimes, tRNA pseudogenes are also found.

Small Nuclear RNA (SnRNA) Genes: Small nuclear RNAs (SnRNAs) are found in abundance in the nuclei of all eukaryotes and represent neither tRNA. nor rRNA. Six SnRNAs, that are usually found, range from 100(U6) to 215(U3) nucleotides in length and are involved in RNA processing through formation of SnRNP (small nuclear ribonucleoproteins). These are encoded by multiple copies of identical genes organised in tandem arrays of repeat units, each SnRNA gene being flanked on either side by spacer DNA ranging from 800 bp to 45,000 bp in length in different organisms.

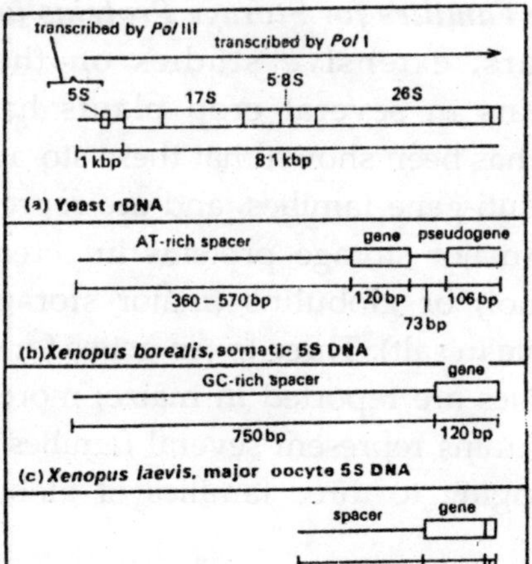

Organisation of 5S DNA (produces 5S RNA for ribosomes) in several organisms; only in yeast it is linked with repeat unit of rDNA in other cases it is independent on a separate chromosome.

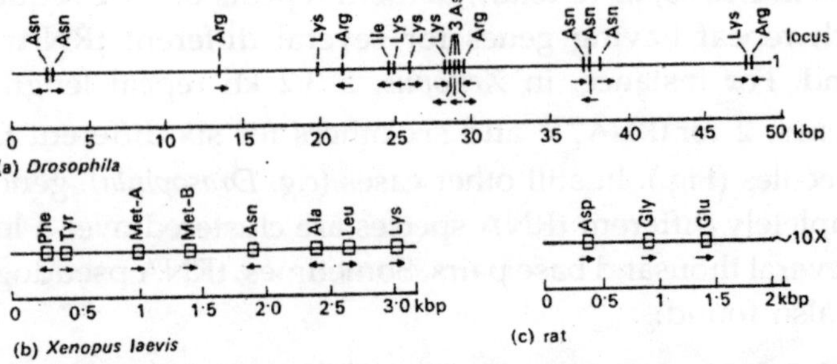

Arrangement of tRNA genes in higher eukaryotes: (a) one of the 50-60 sites on Drosophila chromosomes where tRNA genes are clustered; (b) a 3.18 kilobase-pairs unit from Xenopus DNA, that is repeated about 150 times; (c) rat DNA showing only one of about 10 repeat units found in haploid genome.

An unexpected feature of the DNA that is complementary to SnRNAs is that it consists of many more pseudogenes than the functional genes (10 : 1). For instance in humans, there are 30 genes, for Ul (an SnRNA) on chromosome 1 and 500-1000 pseudogenes distributed throughout the genome.

Multi-gene Families for Storage Proteins in Crop Plants : In recent years, extensive studies on the genetics of storage proteins in several crop plants have also been undertaken. It has been shown that these storage proteins are encoded by multi-gene families, and are represented mainly as prolamins (major storage proteins in cereals—soluble in aqueous alcohol) or globulins (major storage proteins in legumes, soluble in salt). Three to ten genes for each of the ten prolamin families are reported in maize; more than a dozen genes for prolamins represent several families in wheat; and 18 genes belonging to three families of globulin genes are known in pea.

Homologies in genes coding for prolamins and globulins in different crop plants has also been shown. Their multiplicity conveniently meets the demand for rapid synthesis of these proteins in the developing seeds.

Concerted Evolution of Multi-gene Families: The maintenance of a virtual identity among many copies of a multi-gene family, even when located on different chromosomes, suggests that individual members of a gene family can not evolve independently, but rather undergo a concerted evolution. Concerted evolution means that copies of a family evolve as a unit. One may like to know the basis of this concerted evolution in multi-gene families.

In fact, when a large number of copies of the same gene are present, mutation in one or more copies will not have any significant effect on the fitness of the organism, so that we can not explain how will such mutations be eliminated by natural selection; instead we should expect that mutations, particularly those which are neutral should accumulate in course of time. Contrary to this expectation homogeneity is maintained, which has been considered to be a paradox that needs explanation. Experimental and circumstantial evidence suggesting the presence of a mechanism homogenizing the tandemly repeated multi-gene families, is actually available. There are at least two mechanisms that have been proposed:

(i) gene conversion may work at an accelerated rate in a repeated family and may help in homogenisation;

(ii) unequal crossing over may lead to duplications or deletions leading to homogenisation (either mutant member will be deleted or multiply and spread throughout the family).

12

Code of Genes

A recapitulation of the relationship between genes and proteins is desirable for an understanding of the genetic code.

1. All metabolic reactions are catalysed by specific *enzymes*. All enzymes *are proteins*.
2. The action of an enzyme depends upon the *sequence of amino acids* constituting it.
3. The *one-gene one-enzyme hypothesis* proposed by Beadle and Tatum in 1940s states that the synthesis of an enzyme (actually of a polypeptide chain) is controlled by a particular gene.
4. The gene, which is almost always a segment of a DNA strand, *transcribes* an mRNA strand, which in turn *translates* a polypeptide chain.
5. *Messenger RNA* thus acts as an intermediate in conveying information from the sequence of *nucleotides* in DNA to the sequence of *amino acids* in the polypeptide chain (*Sequence Hypothesis*).

6. Each amino acid is specified by a sequence of three bases *(the codon)* on mRNA.
7. Each tRNA molecule has a sequence of three bases *(the anticodon)* which reads a codon of mRNA. Transfer RNA molecules thus serve as *adaptors* in proteins synthesis by reading mRNA codons in a sequence (Crick's *Adaptor Hypothesis).*
8. The relationship between the sequence of bases in DNA | RNA and the sequence of amino acids in a polypeptide chain is called the *genetic code.* The code indicates which codons specify which amino acids.

Amino Acids Involved in Protein Synthesis: About 150 amino acids are found in nature,of which only 20 are specified by the genetic code. Only these 20 amino acids take part in protein synthesis. Among the other amino acids found in proteins are *cystine* and *hydroxyproline. Cystine* is a double amino acid consisting of two *cysteine* units.

It is formed by oxidation which produces a disulphiuc linkage between two cysteine molecules. This disulphide linkage plays an important part in maintaining the tertiary structure of proteins. It is cysteine which is incorporated in the polypeptide chain during protein synthesis. Cystine is then formed as a result of interaction between two cysteine molecules. *Hydroxyproline,* which is particularly found in collagen, is formed by the addition of hydroxyl (OH) group to *proline,* after the latter has been incorporated into the polypeptide chain.

The genes of a cell contain coded information for the maintenance and reproduction of the cell. They direct the arrangement of the 20 types of amino acids into the polypeptide chains of the protein molecules. A polypeptide chain typically contains about 100-300 amino acids, and is formed by specific arrangement of the 20 types of amino acids.

Genetic Code is a Triplet Code: DNA contains four kinds of nucleotides (of A, T, G and C), and proteins are synthesised from 20 different types of amino acids. A basic problem regarding the genetic code was : how many bases of DNA specify one amino acid? In a *singlet code* each base or letter would specify one amino acid.

Only 4 of the 20 types of amino acids would be coded unambiguously by a singlet code (Table). In a two-letter or *doublet* code two bases would specify one amino acid. Here 16 (4 × 4) of the 20 amino acids can be specified, but there would be ambiguous determination of a number of amino acids. A *triplet* or three-letter code was first suggested by the physicist Gamow in 1954.

According to the triplet code three letters or bases specify one amino acid. Thus 64 (4 × 4 × 4) distinct triplets of purine and/or pyrimidine bases determine the 20 amino acids. These triplets have been called *codons.*

Since there are 64 codons and only 20 amino acids it is obvious that there are many more codons than there are amino acids, i.e. the code is *degenerate.* Experimental evidence shows that the code is a triplet one, and that 61 of the 64 codons code for individual amino acids during protein synthesis.

Type of code	*Number of bases in codon*	*Number of codons*	*Ambiguous/ degenerate*
Singlet code	1	4	Ambiguous
Doublret code	2	4 × 4 = 16	Ambiguous
Triplet code	3	4 × 4 × 4 = 64	Degenerate

The Maximum Possible Number of Codons in the Singlet, Doublet and Triplet Codes: A *quadruplet code* would have 4 × 4 × 4 × 4 = 256 codons, and would show even more degeneracy than the triplet code.

Non-overlapping Code

Since the DNA molecule is a long chain of nucleotides it could be read either in an *overlapping* or *non-overlapping* manner. The genetic code could thus be overlapping or non-overlapping. The reading of the code by these two different ways would yield different results. In the *non-overlapping code* six nucleotides would code for *two* amino acids, while in the *overlapping* code up to *four* could be coded (Fig.). In the non-overlapping code each letter is read only once while in the overlapping code it would be read three times, each time as a part of a different word. Mutational changes in one letter would affect only one word in the non-overlapping code white it would affect three words in the overlapping code. Non-overlapping code.

(C, A, T & G are bases.
aal and aa2 are amino acids).
Overlapping code.

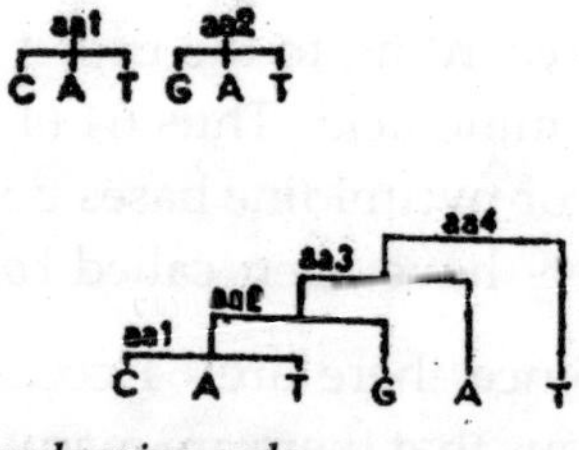

Non-overlapping and overlapping code.

Studies on gene mutations show that *the code is of the non-over lapping type*. In the tobacco mosaic virus (TMV) mutation of one base of the nucleic acid into another results in the alteration of only a single amino acid. Similarly, studies on normal and sickle cell haemoglobins show that a single mutational change results in the substitution of only one amino acid.

Recently it has been shown that in the bacterial virus *ϕ X174* there is a possibility of overlapping of genes (Barrel and co-workers 1976, Sanger *et al*, 1977). Two genes contain the codes for second proteins with different amino acid sequences. Each of the two genes codes for different sequences of amino acids by a frame shift *(overlapping code)* and produces two totally different proteins (see 'Genes within genes', p. 236).

Commaless Code

Is the genetic code read in an uninterrupted manner from one end of the nucleic acid chain to the other ? Or are there bases (commas) between successive codons? A code with commas could be represented as follows (the X represents a base acting as a comma).

UUU X CUC X GUA X UCC X ACC .... Bases

Phe Leu Val Ser Thr .... Amino acids

A mutation resulting in an addition or deletion of a base would affect only one amino acid of the polypeptide chain. The total genetic message would be only slightly changed.

UUU X - UC X GUA X UCC X ACC .... Bases

Phe *Changed aa* Val Ser Thr ....Amino acids

A commaless code would not have the comma bases and can be represented thus:

UUU CUC GUA UCC ACC ....Bases

Phe Leu Val Ser Thr................ Amino acids

In such a code any mutation involving a deletion of a base (—C) would result in a drastic change in the genetic message.

UUU UCG UAU CCA CC .... Bases

Phe *Ser Tyr Pro*...........................Amino acids

The entire series of amino acids following the deletion would change.

All the available evidence indicates that *the code is commaless,* i.e. there are no demarcating signals between codons. The work of Khorana and his associates cited below gives clear evidence of a commaless code. Long synthetic polynucleotides with specific repeating sequences were used for translation of protein chains. Thus the repeating sequence CUCUCU..........

contains the codons CUC (for *leucine*) and UCU (for *serine*). When this sequence is used for translation of proteins, neither amino acid is incorporated into the protein unless the other is also present. This result can only be explained by a commaless triplet code where there would have to be alternate translation of CUC and UCU codons.

Polarity in Code

If a gene is to specify the same protein repeatedly it is essential that the code must be read between fixed start and end points. These points are the *initiation* and the *termination codons*, respectively. It is also essential that the code must be read in a fixed *direction*. In other words the code must have *polarity*. It is obvious that if the code is read in opposite directions it would specify two different proteins, since the codons would have reversed base sequences. Thus if the message given below is read from left to right the first codon, UUG, would specify *leucine*. If read

Codons UUG AUC GUC UCG CCA ACA AGG

→ Leu Ile Val Ser Pro Thr Arg

Val Leu Leu Ala Thr Thr Gly ←

from right to left the codon would become GUU and would specify *valine*. It is thus seen that the sequence of amino acids constituting the protein would undergo a drastic change if the code is read in the opposite direction. The available evidence indicates that the message in mRNA is read in the 5' → 3' direction. The polypeptide chain is synthesised in the N → C direction, i.e. from the *amino* (NH_2) terminal to the *carboxyl* (COOH) terminal.

Codons vs. Anticodons

During translation the codons of mRNA pair with complementary anticodons of tRNA. Since mRNA is read in a polar manner in the 5' → 3' direction the codons are also written in the 5' → 3' direction. Thus the codon AUG is written as 5'AUG3'. The corresponding anticodon on tRNA should therefore be written as 5'CAU3', In such a configuration the first bases of both codon and anticodon would be the ones at the 5' end and third bases at the 3' end.

Base number		1	2	3	
Codon (mRNA)	5'	A	U	G	3'
Anticodon (tRNA)	3'	U	A	C	5'
Base number		3	2	1	

Often, however, the anticodon is written in the 3'→5' direction so as to bring about an easier correlation between the bases of the codon and anticodon. Thus the anticodon for AUG is written as 3' UAC 5' or, more simply, UAC. Here the first letter in the codon is at the 5' end and the first letter of the anticodon at the 3' end.

Primary Codons

The starting amino acid in the synthesis of most protein chains is *methionine* (eukaryotes) or *N-formylmethionine* (prokaryotes). Methionyl or N-formyl methionyl-tRNA specifically binds to *initiation sites* containing the AUG codon. This codon is therefore called the *initiation codon.* Less often, GUG also serves as the initiation codon in bacterial protein synthesis. Normally GUG is the codon for *valine.* In the phage MS2, GUG is the initiation codon for the A protein. GUG has been found to initiate protein synthesis when the normal AUG codon is lost by deletion. However, initiation by GUG is less efficient since it has a lower affinity for fMet-tRNA.

Both AUG and GUG codons show ambiguity in one sense, since each of them codes for two different amino acids. When these two codons are at *initiation positions* of mRNA they code for *N-formyl methionine*. In *internal positions* AUG codes for *methionine* and GUG for *valine*.

Conclusive Codons

Three of the 64 codons do not specify any tRNA. and were hence called *nonsense codons*. These codons are UAG (*amber*), UAA (*ochre*) and UGA (*opal* or *umber*). Since they bring about termination of polypeptide chain synthesis they are also called *termination codons*. UAG was the first termination codon to be discovered. It was named 'amber' after a graduate student named Bernstein (the German for 'amber') who helped in the discovery of a class of mutations. Apparently to give uniformity the other two termination codons were also named after colours.

Termination codons do not code for any amino acids and hence cause termination and release of polypeptide chains. Apparently no tRNA species has anticodons complementary to the termination codons. There are mRNAs with single termination codons and also mRNAs with two successive termination codons (e.g. MS2 coat protein mRNA). Termination codons are not read by any tRNA molecules but by proteins called *release factors*. In *prokaryotes* there are three release factors RF-1, RF-2 and RF-3. RF-1 recognises UAA and UAG, while RF-2 recognises UAA and UGA. RF-3 stimulates RF-1 and RF-2. In *eukaryotes* a single release factor (RF) recognises all three termination codons.

Degenerated Code

As mentioned previously, there are 64 possible codons in a triplet code of which 61 have been shown to code amino acids. Since only 20 amino acids take part in protein synthesis it is obvious that there are many more codons than amino acid types. Except for *tryptophan* and *methionine*, which have a single codon each, all other amino acids involved in protein synthesis have more than one codon. *Phenylalanine, tyro~ sine, histidine, glutamine, asparagine, lysine, aspartic acid, glutamic acid* and *cysteine* have two codons each. *Isoleucine* has three codons. *Valine, proline, threonine, alanine* and *glycine* have four codons each. *Leucine, arginine* and *serine* have six codons each (Table). This variability in the number of codons for different amino acids may at least partially account for the unequal distribution of the different amino acids in protein. In general, the frequency of appearance of amino acids in proteins roughly corresponds to the number of available codons.

Number of Codons Coding for different Aminoacids. Aminoacids in Categories 2-5 are Coded by more than one Codon. Such Codons are Called Degenerate

	Amino Acids	*Number of codons*
1.	Tryptophan, methionine	1
2.	Phenylalanine, tyrosine, histidine, glutamine, asparagine	2
	lysine, aspartic acid, glutamic acid, cysteine	2
3.	Isoleucine	3
4.	Valine, proline, threonine, alanine, glycine	4
5.	Leucine, arginine, serine	6

Wobble Model

The triplet code is a degenerate one with many more codons than the number of amino acid types coded. An explanation for this degeneracy is provided by the 'wobble hypothesis' proposed by Crick (1966). Since there are 61 codons specifying amino acids, the cell should contain 61 different tRNA molecules, each with a different anticodon. Actually, however, the number of tRNA molecule types discovered is much less than 61. This implies that the anticodons of some tRNAs read more than one codon on mRNA.

According to the wobble hypothesis only the first two positions of a triplet codon on mRNA have a precise pairing with the bases of the tRNA anticodon. The pairing of the third position bases of the codon may be ambiguous, and varies according to the nucleotide present in this position. Thus a single tRNA type is able to recognise two or more codons differing only in the third base. The anticodon UCG of *serine tRNA* recognises two codons, AGC and AGU. The bonding between UCG and AGC follows the usual Watson-Crick pairing pattern. In UCG. AGU pairing, however, hydrogen bonding takes place between G and U. This is a departure from the usual Watson-Crick pairing mechanism where G pairs with C and A with U. Such interaction between the third bases is referred to as *'wobble pairing'*.

mRNA codons (serine)	5'	AGC	3'	5'	AGU	3'
tRNA anticodon	3'	UCG	5'	3'	UCG	5'

The degeneracy of the code is not random. Mostly the different codons for a particular amino acid have the same first two letters (*leucine, serine* and *arginine* are exceptions). Thus the first two letters of all the four codons for *valine* are GU and for *alanine* GC.

1st base in the codon	Second base in the codon: U	C	A	G	3rd base in the codon
U	UUU Phenylalanine	UCU Serine	UAU Tyrosine	UGU Cysteine	U
	UUC Phenylalanine	UCC Serine	UAC Tyrosine	UGC Cysteine	C
	UUA Leucine	UCA Serine	UAA TERMINATION (3) (ocher)	UGA TERMINATION (3) (opal)	A
	UUG Leucine (2)	UCG Serine	UAG TERMINATION (3) (amber)	UGG Tryptophan	G
C	CUU Leucine	CCU Proline	CAU Histidine	CGU Arginine	U
	CUC Leucine	CCC Proline	CAC Histidine	CGC Arginine	C
	CUA Leucine	CCA Proline	CAA Glutamine	CGA Arginine	A
	CUG Leucine	CCG Proline	CAG Glutamine	CGG Arginine	G
A	AUU Isoleucine	ACU Threonine	AAU Asparagine	AGU Serine	U
	AUC Isoleucine	ACC Threonine	AAC Asparagine	AGC Serine	C
	AUA Isoleucine	ACA Threonine	AAA Lsyine	AGA Arginine	A
	AUG Methionine (1) (INITIATION)	ACG Threonine	AAG Lsyine	AGG Arginine	G
G	GUU Valine	GCU Alanine	GAU Aspartic acid	GGU Glycine	U
	GUC Valine	GCC Alanine	GAC Aspartic acid	GGC Glycine	C
	GUA Valine	GCA Alanine	GAA Glutamic acid	GGA Glycine (4)	A
	GUG Valine (2)	GCG Alanine	GAG Glutamic acid	GGG Glycine	G

The genetic code.

(The numbers in brackets refer to the notes for Table).

Notes for Table

1. *Methionine* is the starting amino acid of eukaryote polypeptides, and *N-formyl methionine* of 'bacterial

polypeptides. The codon for these aminoacids is AUG, which is called the *initiation codon* because it starts protein synthesis,

2. *N-formyl methionine* is probably also coded by UUG and GUG, which then also function as *initiation codons.*
3. UAA, UAG and UGA called ochre, amber and opal, respectively were called *'nonsense' codons* since they do not code for any aimno acid. They are responsible for signalling the termination of the polypeptide chain, and are therefore called *termination codons or stop codons.* They are read by specific proteins called *release factors,* and not by any tRNAs.
4. *GGA* probably also codes for *glutamic acid.* When a codon codes for more than one amino acid the code is said to be *ambiguous.*

When only two codons specify an amino acid the third letters of the codons are either *both purincs* or *both pyrimidines:* never one purine and one pyrimidine.

Third Base

	Pyrimidine	*Purine*	*Pyrimidine*	*Purine*	
Codons	UUU	UUA	CAU	CAA	Watson-Crick pairing
	UUC	UUG	CAC	CAG	Wobble pairing
Amino acids	Phe	Leu	His	Glu	
Anticodons	AAA	AAU	GUA	GUU	

It is possible to predict the minimum number of tRNAs required to translate the different codons specifying a particular amino acid. The amino acid *leucine* is specified by six codons: UUA, UUG, CUU, CUC, CUA and CUG. The first two letters of two codons are UU and of four codons CU. Hence at least two different tRNAs are required, since the first two letters of a codon do not have wobble pairing with the anticodon.

Of the four codons having CU two (CUU and CUC) have *pyrimidines* as their third bases and two (CUA and CUG) have *purines.* Hence they cannot be read by the same anticodon, because the purine of the anticodon can only pair with a pyrimidine and *vice versa.*

The CU-codons must therefore be read by at least two different anticodons. Thus *at least three codons* are required to read to anticodons for leucine.

Presumably the anticodons AUU reads UUA and UAG, GAA reads CUU and CUC, and GAU reads CUA and CUG. It will be seen that each anticodon has Watson-Crick pairing with third base of one codon, and wobble pairing with the third base of the other codon.

Third Base

	Pnrine		*Pyrimidine*		*Purine*	
Codons	*DUA*	UUG	CUU	CUC	*CVA*	CUG
Anticodons	AAU	*AAU*	GAA	GAA	GAU	*GAU*
Type of pairing	WCP	WP	WCP	WP	WCP	WP

WCP=Watson-Crick pairing with anticodon. WP =Wobble pairing with anticodon. The six codons of leucine and their pairing with three types of anticodons.

The anticodon of certain tRNAs contains *inosine* (I), a deamination product of adenosine. Inosine closely resembles G and would thus be expected to pair with C. It is found to bond with C, A or U.

Thus a tRNA with its anticodon having I in the wobble position would be able to pair with three codons having C, A or U in the third position. *Isoleucine* is the only amino acid to have three codons, these being AUC/AUC and AUA. *A* tRNA molecule having the anticodon UAI would be able to pair with all these three codons (Fig.).

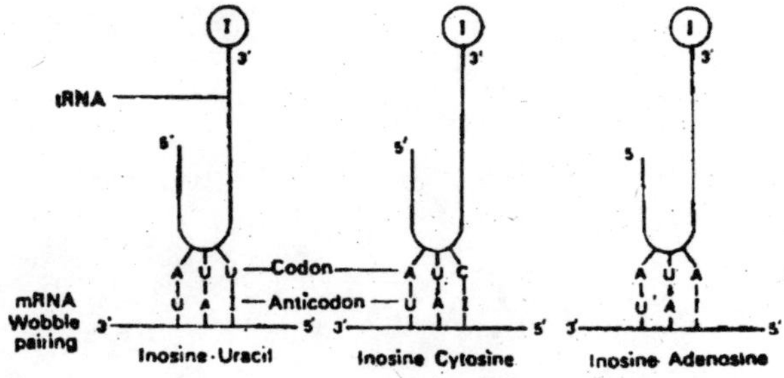

Wobble pairing of inosine with uracil cytosine andadenine.

Codons for isoleucine	AUU	AUC	*ADA*
Anticodon	UAI	UAI	UAI

I cannot pair with G. Had it been able to do so the anticodon UAI would have also paired with AUG, the initiation codon specifying *Methionine.*

Wobble pairing takes place in only certain combinations. Three types have been proposed: (i) U in the wobble position of the tRNA anticodon can pair with A or G of the mRNA codon, (ii) G can pair with U or C and (iii) I can pair with A, U or C.

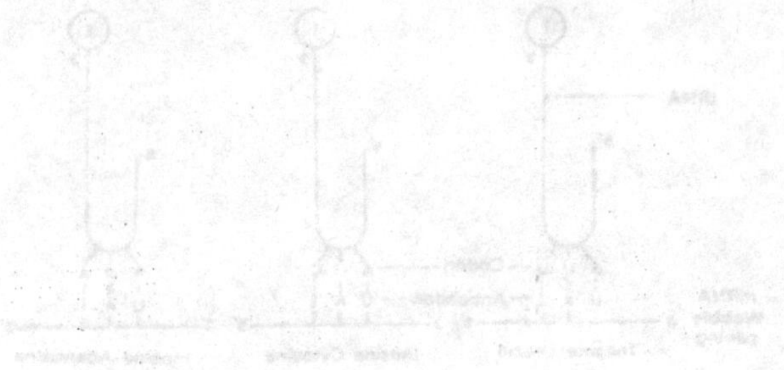

Bibliography

Abbas, A.K, A.H. Lichtman and, J.S. Pober : *Cellular and Molecular Immunology,* Saunders, Philadelphia, 1999.

Ameisen, J. C. : *Tissue Culture,* Oxford, New York, 2000.

Anderson, S. : *Cell Biology,* Oxford University Press, London, 1981.

Atkins, J. F. : *Tissue Culture: an Introduction,* Oxford, New York, 1996.

Auerbach, C. : *Mutation Research: Problems, Results and Perspectives,* Chapman and Hall, London, 2002.

Baker, T.A. : *DNA Replication,* Freeman, New York, 2002.

Beale, G.H. : *Cellular Control Mechanisms and Cancer,* Oxford, New York, 2002.

Becker, W.M. and D.W. Deamer : *The World of the Cell,* Benjamin-Cummings, Redwood City, 2000.

Benjamin, Lewin : *Genes,* Oxford University Press, New York, 2000.

Bennett, R. H. : *Transcription, Processing and Editing in Plant Mitochondria,* Oxford, New York, 1992.

Bittar, E.E. : *Cell Biology in Medicine,* John Wiley, New York, 1999.

Branden, C. and Tooze, J. : *Introduction to Cell Biology,* Garland, New York, 1991.

Court, D. : *Regulatory Sequences Involved in the Promotion and Termination of RNA Transcription,* Cambridge, New York, 2003.

Darnell, J. E. : *Molecular Cell Biology,* Scientific American Books, New York, 1995.

Das, A. : *Control of Transcription Termination,* Routledge, New York, 1993.

Demidov, V. V. : *PNA and LNA throw Light on DNA, Trends,* Oxford, New York, 2003.

DeRobertis, E.D.P. : *Cell Biology,* Waverly Pvt. Ltd., New Delhi, 1988.

DuPraw, E. J. : *Cell and Molecular Biology,* Academic Press, New York, 1969.

Ebby, S. R. : *Non Coding RNA Genes and Modern RNA,* Oxford, New York, 2001

Edlin, G. : *Human Genetics : A Modern Synthesis,* Jones & Bartlett Pub., Boston, 1990.

Ellis, R. J. : *Chloroplast Protein Synthesis,* Oxford, New York, 1975.

Fincham, J.R.S. : *Genetic Complementation,* Benjamin, New York, 1999.

Fournier, M.J. : *The Small Nucleolar RNAs,* MacMillan, London, 1995.

Friedberg, E. C. : *Relationships Between DNA Repair and Transcription,* Oxford, New York, 1996.

Gilbert, W. and B. Muller : *Isolation of the Lac Repressor,* Oxford, New York, 1966.

Gilham, N. W. : *Genetic Analysis of the Chloroplast and Mitochondrial Genomes,* Oxford, New York, 1974.

Glick, B. and G. Schatz : *Import of Proteins into Mitochondria,* Oxford, New York, 1991.

Gray, M. W. : *The Evolutionary Origin of Organelles*, Oxford, New York, 1989.

Grunstein, M. : *Histones as Regulators of Genes*, Oxford, New York, 1992.

Gupta, P. K. : *Cell Biology*, Rastogi Publications, Meerut, 2000.

Hadjiolov, A. A. : *The Nucleolus and Ribosome Biogenesis*, Oxford, New York, 1985.

Henikoff, S. : *Cell Biology : A Reference Manual*, MIT Press, Cambridge, 2002.

Hoagland, M. G. : *The Present Status of the Adaptor Hypothesis*, MacMillan, London, 1959.

Holley, R. W. : *Structure of a Ribonucleic Acid*, McGraw Hill, London, 2002.

Hunt, T. : *The Cell Cycle*, Oxford University Press, Oxford, 2002.

Ingram, V. : *The Biosynthesis of Macromolecules*, Benjamin, New York, 2001.

Jacobson, M. : *Developmental Neurobiology*, Plenum Press, New York, 2002.

Jukes, T. H. : *Mitochondrial Codes and Evolution*, Oxford, New York, 2000.

Kaguni, L. S. : *Eukaryotic DNA Polymerase-primase : Structure, Mechanism and Function*, MacMillan, London, 1999.

Kaziro, Y: *Structure and Function of Signal Transducing GTP Binding Proteins*, Blackwell, London, 2001.

Kendrew, J. C. : *The Three-dimensional Structure of a Protein Molecule*, Sinauer, New York, 1991

Kramer, A. :*The Structure and Function of Proteins Involved in Mammalian Pre-mRNA Splicing*, Grandada, New York, 2001.

Kurland, C. G. : *Structure and Function of the Bacterial Ribosomes*, Oxford, New York, 2000.

Lehninger, A. L. : *Cell Biology*, Academic Press, New York, 2001

McKnight, S. L. : *Molecular Zippers in Gene Regulation*, Princeton, New York, 2002.

Merrick, W. C. : *Overview : Mechanism of Translation Initiation in Eukaryotes*, Longman, London, 2001.

Moore, P. B. : *Molecular Mimicry in Protein Synthesis*, Cambridge, London, 2002.

Noller, H. F. : *Ribosomol RNA and Translation*, Oxford, New York, 1999.

Olson, R. E. : *Enzymatic Synthesis of DNA*, John Wiley, New York, 2001.

Owen, L. : *DNA Synthesis*, Freeeman, San Francisco, 2001.

Pardee, A. B. : *Molecular Basis of Biological Regulation: Origins of Feedback Inhibition and Allostery*, Arnold, London, 2003.

Paszkowski, J. : *DNA and Histone Methylation in Plants*, MacMillan, London, 2002.

Razin, A. and A. D. Riggs : *DNA Methylation and Gene Function*, Longman, New York, 2002.

Reinbcrg, D. : *Common Themes in Assembly and Function of Eukaryotic Transcription Complexes*, MacMillan, London, 2002.

Rich, A. and S. H. Kim : *The Three Dimensional Structure of Transfer RNA*, Oxford, New York, 1999.

Robertson, M. : *RNA Processing : the Post-RNA World*, Oxford, New York, 1999.

Sauer, R. T. : *Transcription Factors : Structural Families and Principles of DNA Recognition*, Printice Hall, London, 1993.

Schmid, M. B. : *Structure and Function of the Bacterial Chromosome*, Granada, London, 1990.

Stryer, L. : *Cell Biology*, W.H. Freeman & Co., New York, 2002.

Temin, H. M. : *RNA Directed DNA Synthesis,* MacGraw-Hill, New York, 2002.

Threadgold, L.T. : *The Infrastructure of Animal Cell,* Pergamon Press, London, 1999.

Turner, B. M. : *Histone Acetylation and Control of Gene Expression,* MacMillan, London, 2002.

Ulrich, B. : *Mechanism and Regulation of Eukaryotic Protein Synthesis,* Oxford, New York, 2002.

Uptain, S. M. : *Basic Mechanisms of Transcript Elongation and its Regulation,* MacMillan, London, 1997.

Voinnet, O. : *RNA Silencing : Small RNAs as Ubiquitous Regulators of Gene Expression,* MacMillan, London, 2002.

Walbot, V. : *Structure of Plant Mitochondrial Genomes,* John Wiley, London, 1992.

Wallace, D. C. : *Diseases of the Mitochondrial DNA,* Blackwell, New York, 2002.

Wang, T. S. F. : *Eukaryotic DNA Polymerases,* MacMillan, London, 2002.

Wilkins, M. H. F. : *Physical Studies of the Molecular Structure of Deoxyribose Nucleic Acid and Nucleoprotein,* MacMillan, London, 2002.

Woese, C. R. : *The Genetic Code : The Molecular Basis for Genetic Expression,* Harper & Row, New York, 2003.

Wuthrich, K. : *A Hand Book of Cell Biology,* Oxford, New York, 2001.

Yanofsky, C. : *Introduction Tissue Culture,* Oxford, New York, 2001.

Yarus, M. : *Translational Efficiency of Transfer RNAs,* Oxford, New York, 2002.

Zetka, M. : *History of Tissue Culture,* Oxford, New York, 2002.

Index

H

I

J

K

L

M

N

O

P

Q

R

S

T

U

V

W

X

❑❑❑

20/10/02